T0254823

Lecture Notes of the Institute for Computer Sciences, Social Informatics and Telecommunications Engineering 314

More information about this series at http://www.springer.com/series/8197

Nuno M. Garcia · Ivan Miguel Pires ·
Rossitza Goleva (Eds.)

IoT Technologies for HealthCare

6th EAI International Conference, HealthyIoT 2019
Braga, Portugal, December 4–6, 2019
Proceedings

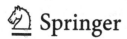

Springer

Editors
Nuno M. Garcia 🆔
Department of Computer Science
University of Beira Interior
Covilha, Portugal

Ivan Miguel Pires 🆔
University of Beira Interior
Covilha, Portugal

Rossitza Goleva 🆔
New Bulgarian University
Sofia, Bulgaria

ISSN 1867-8211   ISSN 1867-822X (electronic)
Lecture Notes of the Institute for Computer Sciences, Social Informatics
and Telecommunications Engineering
ISBN 978-3-030-42028-4   ISBN 978-3-030-42029-1 (eBook)
https://doi.org/10.1007/978-3-030-42029-1

This Springer imprint is published by the registered company Springer Nature Switzerland AG
The registered company address is: Gewerbestrasse 11, 6330 Cham, Switzerland

Preface

The 6th EAI International Conference on IoT Technologies for HealthCare (HealthyIoT 2019) took place in the beautiful town of Braga, Portugal, on December 4–6, 2019, under the umbrella of the 5th annual Smart City 360° Summit. The event was endorsed by the European Alliance for Innovation, an international professional community-based organization devoted to the advancement of innovation in the field of ICT.

HealthyIoT 2019 was the 6th edition of an international scientific event series dedicated to Internet of Things (IoT) and Healthcare. IoT, as a paradigm leveraging a set of existing and emerging technologies, notions, and services, can provide many solutions to delivery of electronic healthcare, patient care, and medical data management. HealthyIoT aims to bring together technology experts, researchers, industry professionals, and international authorities contributing towards the design, development, and deployment of healthcare solutions based on IoT technologies, standards, and procedures.

The technical program of HealthyIoT 2019 consisted of 10 full papers in oral presentation sessions at the main workshop tracks. The papers submitted and presented during the workshop cover many health sensors and systems technologies, applications, and services, as well as solutions. Sensor data synchronization in the IoT environment was presented as the devices from different producers generate data in different formats and often are not capable to timestamp the values after measurements. Important implementation for infants motricity measurement was shown. Photoplethysmogram (PPG) signal processing is another hot topic related to the blood pressure measurement. A measurement of PPG in real-time especially during intense physical activity is applied for studying the physical condition of the people. Electromyography (EMG) sensor embedded into textile was developed to control the functions of the prosthesis. Important design of a smart mechatronic system to combine garments for blind people was also demonstrated.

IoT for health applications and solutions presented more complex approaches aiming to create market ready devices and software. Smartwatch blood pressure measurement using PPG signal and physiological features was proposed. Smartphone based monitoring for automatic eating control through Wi-Fi presented an interesting approach for lonely people under social monitoring. The solution called SocialBike quantified data from physical activity. Nice tool assisting the radiologists in X-ray diagnostics supports the everyday work in the screening clinics. Wireless medical systems for forensic was shown. Smart home assisting services through an IoT-based healthcare ecosystem was demonstrated.

Coordination with the steering chair, Imrich Chlamtac, as well as valuable support from Nuno M. Garcia, Aleksandar Jevremovic, Nuno Pombo, Susanna Spinsante, Francisco Floréz-Revuelta, Ivan Pires, Kristina Lappyova, Miguel Castelo-Branco,

Hugo Silva, and Henriques Zacarias was essential for the success of the workshop. We sincerely appreciate their constant work and guidance.

We strongly believe that the HealthyIoT 2019 workshop provided a good forum for all researcher, developers, and practitioners to discuss all science and technology aspects that are relevant to smart health. We also expect that the future HealthyIoT workshops will be as successful and stimulating, as indicated by the contributions presented in this volume.

December 2019

Imrich Chlamtac
Nuno M. Garcia
Aleksandar Jevremovic
Nuno Pombo
Susanna Spinsante

Organization

Steering Committee

Imrich Chlamtac   University of Trento, Italy

Organizing Committee

General Chair

Nuno M. Garcia   University of Beira Interior, Portugal

General Co-chairs

Aleksandar Jevremovic   Singidunum University, Serbia
Nuno Pombo   University of Beira Interior, Portugal

TPC Chair

Susanna Spinsante   Marche Polytechnic University, Italy

Sponsorship and Exhibit Chair

Miguel Castelo-Branco   University of Beira Interior, Portugal

Local Chair

Ivan Pires   University of Beira Interior, Portugal

Workshop Chair

Francisco Floréz-Revuelta   University of Alicante, Spain

Publicity and Social Media Chair

Hugo Silva   Instituto de Telecomunicações, Portugal

Publications Chair

Rossitza Goleva   New Bulgarian University, Bulgaria

Web Chair

Henriques Zacarias   University of Beira Interior, Portugal

Conference Manager

Kristina Lappyova   EAI

Technical Program Committee

An Braeken	Vrije Universiteit Brussel, Belgium
Angelica Poli	Marche Polytechnic University, Italy
Ciprian Dobre	National Institute for Research and Development in Informatics, Romania
Constandinos X. Mavromoustakis	University of Nicosia, Cyprus
Eftim Zdravevski	Saints Cyril and Methodius University, North Macedonia
Emmanuel Conchon	University of Limoges, France
Ennio Gambi	Marche Polytechnic University, Italy
Igor Bisio	University of Genoa, Italy
Ivan Ganchev	University of Limerick, Ireland
Ivan Pires	University of Beira Interior, Portugal
Lina Xu	University College Dublin, Ireland
Lorenzo Palma	Marche Polytechnic University, Italy
Manuela Montangero	University of Modena, Italy
Marko Sarac	Singidunum University, Serbia
Milan Tair	Singidunum University, Serbia
Pau Climent-Pérez	University of Alicante, Spain
Saša Adamović	Singidunum University, Serbia
Silvia Mirri	University of Bologna, Italy
Virginie Felizardo	University of Beira Interior, Portugal

Contents

IoT for Health Sensors and Systems

Sensor Data Synchronization in a IoT Environment for Infants Motricity Measurement

Simone Sguazza[1], Alessandro Puiatti[1], Sandra Bernaschina[1],
Francesca Faraci[1], Gianpaolo Ramelli[3], Vincenzo D'Apuzzo[2],
Emmanuelle Rossini[1], and Michela Papandrea[1(✉)]

[1] University of Applied Sciences and Arts of Southern Switzerland (SUPSI),
Manno, Switzerland
{simone.sguazza,alessandro.puiatti,sandra.bernaschina,francesca.faraci,
emmanuelle.rossini,michela.papandrea}@supsi.ch
[2] Centro Pediatrico del Mendrisiotto (CPM), Mendrisio, Switzerland
[3] Ente Ospedaliero Cantonale (EOC), Bellinzona, Switzerland

Abstract. Sensor data synchronization is a critical issue in the Internet of Things environments. In general, when a measurement environment includes different independent devices, it is paramount to ensure a global data consistency to a reference timestamp. Additionally, sensor nodes clocks are typically affected by environmental effects and by energy constraints which generate clock drifts. In this work, we present a specific Internet of Things architecture composed by seven Inertial Measurement Unit nodes, three Raspberry Pi 3, three video cameras and a laptop. In specific, we present an off-line data-driven synchronization solution which handles data of different nature and sampled at different frequencies. The solution solves both the data synchronization issue and the data-time alignment due to clock drift problems. The proposed methodology has been implemented and deployed within a measurement context involving infants (from 8 to 15 months old), within the scope of the AutoPlay project, whose goal is the analysis of infants ludic motricity data in order to possibly anticipate the identification of neurodevelopmental disorders.

Keywords: IoT system · Sensor data synchronization · Activity inference · NDD early detection · Healthy youth · Infants · Play

1 Introduction

The AutoPlay project [3] consists in the design and implementation of an IoT solution as an application for supporting pediatricians in the early diagnosis of neuro-developmental disorders. In particular, AutoPlay investigates the development of toys manipulation patterns in the very small children ludic behavior (less than 2 years old). The infants manipulation analysis results are then exploited in order to build infant ludic behavioural models, and to create a prediction model able to support pediatricians in the identification of atypical infant ludic behaviour, which could be related to social problems or neurodevelopmental disorders.

The very final objective of AutoPlay is reaching a social systematic change on how ludic behavior is observed, analysed and considered for evaluating and identifying early signs of neurodevelopmental disorders and social problems. This will allow the anticipation of the diagnosis and the necessary therapy, hence increasing the opportunity for a better quality of life.

In this work we describe the IoT solution exploited for an initial pilot study, aimed at creating a first database of infants ludic behavioural data. The data collected during this pilot consists in video recordings and inertial measurements data. In particular, in this work we present the preprocessing analysis performed over the collected data, and in particular the designed and implemented data synchronization procedure, necessary for quantifying and handling the non constant time shift between the chock of the different data sources. The main goal of the presented data synchronization procedure is to generate a reliable and usable dataset which can be subsequently applied to a machine learning analysis for manipulation activity inference.

The rest of the paper is structured as follows. Section 2 briefly summarizes the state of the art approaches for sensor data synchronization in IoT environments. Section 3 presents the materials and methodologies applied for the AutoPlay project and the related design and implementation of the IoT system architecture. Section 4 is the main part of the paper: it provides a presentation of the pre-processing task and related issues, and provides a detailed description of the implemented two/steps synchronization solution. Finally, Sect. 5 presents a final discussion on the presented work, future works and possible alternative solutions.

2   Related Works

Time synchronization is a critical issue in Wireless Sensor Networks (WSN) and Internet of Things (IoT) environments. In general, when a measurement environment includes different independent devices, it is necessary to ensure data consistency to a global reference timestamp: all data captured from different devices, measuring events at the same time, should have the same timestamp. A logical synchronization approach (i.e., the Lamport algorithm for ordering events happened in a distributed environment) does not solve our issue. What we need to identify is a global reference clock, and to synchronize all the heterogeneous sampling devices to it, with a precision in the order of ms. Additionally, we also need to compensate the clock drifts of each sensor nodes, due to environmental effects (i.e., fluctuations in temperature, pressure, humidity) and energy constraints (i.e., limited power resources).

There are different solutions developed for the WSN, where the synchronization procedure is performed by means of wireless messages exchange between pairs of devices [4], or broadcasted to the network [2,8], where the content of the message consists in the actual global timestamp [5,7,12]. Skiadopoulosa et al. [11] presents an approach slightly different from the traditional ones for WSN which induces negligible extra overhead, in fact it does not require extra messages and re-synchronization procedures for handling the clock drift problem: in their approach, data measurements is synchronized instead of node clocks.

These approaches require the establishment of a wireless network between sensor devices as a mesh (all the sensors devices are connected through neighbor nodes) or as a star (each sensor device is connected to a central node, typically a master node).

Traditional data synchronization strategies cannot be applied in many IoT contexts, where sensor devices have intermittent or no connectivity to the network and have limited power resources. There exist different solutions which implement real-time data synchronization [10], or which requires data streaming, and solutions which simply tolerate un-synchronized data. Other synchronization approaches are only based on sensor data and are performed off-line. Luckac et al. [9] present an approach relying on regularly occurring events and a model of the event propagation to allow correction of the time information. This solution is limited in that it requires a known regularly occurring seismic event. Harashima et al. present a synchronization solution assisted by environmental signals [6]. The environmental signals being measured are used as an additive noise that synchronizes the sensors. Because it is expected that the sensors in a limited range will see the same environmental signals, these signals can be used to aid the synchronization. Bettet et al. presents a similar synchronization procedure [1], where the communication between sensors is not required, and it can handle heterogeneous devices.

The technique proposed in this work allows for time synchronization between heterogeneous sensor devices, without the necessity of communication between them. The synchronization is performed off line, allowing the devices to reserve their power resources for the sampling task. The proposed approach is similar to already existing approaches because based on the presence of a reference synchronization event measured by all the devices at the same time. However, differently from the other approaches, it implements a supervised procedure for the identification of the time shift: it maximizes the proximity between the sensors aggregated data signals and a ground truth signal, and measures the clock shifts from the result of the optimization procedure. The usage of the aggregated signal increases the accuracy of the synchronization, which is in the order of milliseconds. The proposed approach works well for environments with multiple sensor devices. If the number of devices is too large, a dynamic device sampling procedure is required for ensuring the procedure scalability.

3   Materials and Data Collection Architecture

The focus of AutoPlay is to understand the way children use toys, in order to detect infants atypical behavioural patterns. To achieve this goal we identified a set of toys belonging to the main sensory-motor classes of play: mouthing, simple manipulation, functional, relational, and functional-relational. More in particular, with the support of a professional toy designer [1] we developed the AutoPlay toys-kit, composed by: a ball, a doll and a spoon, 3 cubes, and a car (Fig. 1).

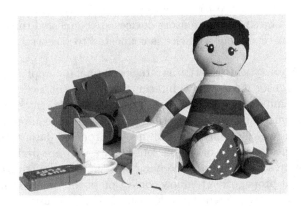

Fig. 1. AutoPlay toys kit

Each toy embeds one 9 DoF IMU (9 Degrees of Freedom Inertial Measurement Unit) sensor node that collects:

- 3D-acceleration data,
- 3D-gyroscope data,
- 3D-magnitude data.

The employed device is the Shimmer3 IMU Unit. The car includes also two rotary encoders attached to the sensor node itself, which are used to measure the movements and directions of the car's wheels (independently of the movement of the car main body).

The IMU sampling frequency is $f_{data} = 100.21$ Hz for all the toys except the car, whose sampling frequency is $f_{data} = 504.12$ Hz. The sampling frequency of the car has been set in order to be able to identify complete wheels rotations (the used rotary encoder is a mechanical encoder with 24 pulses per revolution).

While a child is playing with the toys data are collected locally by the embedded sensors and stored within the sensor node micro-SD card. At the end of each playing session, data are downloaded on a central repository and prepared for the following off-line analysis.

The data collected by sensors are used for the identification of the toy movements. This information is directly correlated to the manipulation activities performed by the infant, thus allowing us to analyze the infant ludic behaviour.

---

[1] Pepe Hiller http://www.pepehiller.com/.

We collect also video recordings of each infant's play session at 25 fps (frames per seconds). These recordings are collected in order to have ground truth (GT) data for the manipulation activities performed by infants. All videos are visualized and used for the creation of corresponding video logs (Fig. 2): each activity performed by the infant during a video recording (playing session) is logged as a row in a log file, which specifies the name of the activity (*Activity*) (from a list of micro-activities initially identified with the support of a clinician), the name of the involved toy (*Toy*), the relative time of the activity within the video in frames (*Frame start* and *Frame and*), the camera from which the activity is visualized and logged, and a categorical value specifying if the activity is seemingly unintentional (*N*) or performed as a consequence of a stimulus from an adult person, the educator (*E*). The timestamp of the video recording is stored as meta-data, and used to keep track of the global timestamp of each activity. The log data is anonymised, in the sense that there is no connection between the collected data and the corresponding playing infant.

The log files generated from the collected videos are used as digital target data, for subsequently training a machine learning model for inferring *infant ludic manipulation activities*.

N o E ?	Activity	Toy	Frame start	Frame end	Cam1	Cam2	Cam3
N	Hit	EV	1012	1051		x	
N	Hit	EV	1054	1075		x	
	Take	EB	1223	1244		x	
	Hold	EB	1245	2346		x	
N	Hit	EA	1567	1575		x	
	Hit	PA	1583	1587		x	
	Roll	PA	1588	1609		x	
N	Hit	CU	1615	1627		x	
N	Hit	EA	1629	1634		x	
	Turn	EB	2153	2215		x	
	Support	EB	2347	2361		x	
N	Hit	EB	2444	2457		x	
N	Hit	EA	2460	2467		x	

Fig. 2. Ground truth log file example

3.1   Architecture

In order to collect manipulation data, we created an ad-hoc Internet of Things Measuring Environment. The networked devices involved in the measurement process are listed below.

1. Three cameras which record the infant activities from different angles. The cameras are located at a distance less than 2 m form the playing area. Their position, with respect to the center of the playing area, is equally distributed in order to be able to visualize all the movements performed by the infant. Each camera is an ad-hoc module applied to a Raspberry Pi 3 Model B.

2. A laptop which is wired connected to the cameras through a switch. The laptop is an interface for the person which manages the playing measurement sessions (the educator). It is used as Network Time Protocol (NTP) server to synchronize the clock of each raspberry device, to remotely access one of the raspberry devices performing a server role (for starting and stopping the video recording for all the cameras), and to collect and store the recorded videos.

3. An IMU sensor node per each toy within the AutoPlay toys-kit.

This ad-hoc environment has been deployed within two local kindergartens in Tessin (Switzerland). The data collection pilot lasted for 15 months and involved 24 infants in the age of 8 to 15 months. The study was conducted in accordance with the Declaration of Helsinki and written consent was provided by all participants families. The study was reviewed and approved by the competent ethics committee (Swiss Ethical Committee of Kanton Tessin, ref. PB 2016-00056) before the start of participants inclusions.

In order to protect infant privacy, the laptop and the raspberry Pi involved in the study, do not have access to the Internet. All sensitive data (video recording, infants demographics and IMU data) are not transmitted via wireless. This particular settings have been decided in accordance with the Swiss Ethical Committee. All the devices wire-connected (within the measurement LAN) are synchronized with each other. A schema of the wired measuring environment is provided in Fig. 3.

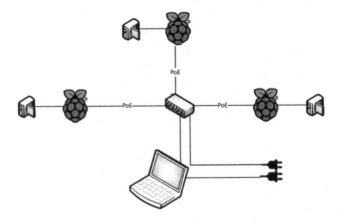

Fig. 3. Measuring environment LAN

The sensor nodes are independent of the other IoT devices. During the described pilot study we tested two possible configurations:

1. sensor nodes synchronized with the measurement LAN by means of BLE (Bluetooth Low Energy) communication with the laptop (data-time synchronization is performed before the video-data collection);

2. sensor nodes completely independent of the sensor LAN during the measurement sessions, the synchronization between the recorded videos and the data collected is performed later on, during the preprocessing analysis.

Details about the two solutions are described in Sect. 4.

4   Methodology

Within the presented architecture, the sensor nodes and the video cameras are independent from each other, generating then a synchronization issue in the collected data. In this paragraph we are going to describe how we handled the synchronization issue between the videos recorded and the sensors collected data. As described in Sect. 3, we implemented two configuration for the sensor data collection. In a first configuration we established a BLE connection between the laptop and each sensor device: the connection allowed the timestamp synchronization (the employed sensor does not have a real-time clock), the sampling frequency configuration, and the sampling session management (start-stop sampling commands). With this measurement configuration, the collected data are already synchronized with the videos recorded by the cameras.

In the second configuration, all the sensor devices are configured and synchronized with each other before the measurement session, but they are not synchronized with the rest of the IoT devices. In this case a synchronization between the video recordings and the sensor collected data is required, and performed offline, during the data preprocessing phase.

The first approach would be the preferable one, because it requires less preprocessing actions. However we opted for the second approach, because even if it requires a synchronization pre-processing procedure, it ensure the absence of data loss, which is indeed very frequent with the first approach. In fact, the BLE communication had reliability issues within our pilot measurement environment. The laptop was not always able to reach all the sensor nodes and the sampling sessions was not always starting when necessary, causing a considerable loss of data.

Within the context of our pilot, data loss is an important negative aspect compared to the increased pre-processing computational effort. The limited availability of infants and families giving their consent for the data collection, and the difficult selection procedure of the appropriate moment during the day for the infant playing sessions, gives a greater value to the actual presence of collected data, even if this data require a pre-processing procedure.

In order to implement the second approach, within the measuring environment, an adult person responsible for the playing sessions (typically a kindergarten educator) had to manually start and stop the sampling procedure on each device. The toys have been designed in such a way that the start/stop sampling button was easily reachable, without completely disassembling the toy (Fig. 4). At the same time, the toys have been designed in such a way that the sampling button was not reachable by an infant.

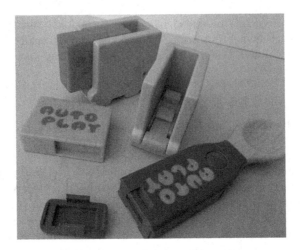

Fig. 4. AutoPlay toys plug details

Additionally, for both configurations, a second phase data-time alignment is required, in order to handle sensor related clock drift issues.

4.1 Sensor Data Synchronization

As explained above, in order to analyze the collected data, an important step is the timestamp synchronization between the recorded videos and the sensors data. The main goal of this task is to identify the *time shift* between them in order to align the sensors data with the ground truth videos.

Additionally, there exist a not negligible clock drift in the collected data, which requires a two-steps synchronization procedure:

1. identification of the overall synchronization *time shift*;
2. perform a per-measurement post-synchronization data-time alignment.

For the synchronization task, we start from the assumption that all the devices timestamp are synchronized to the actual date and time of the day: the synchronization time shift we are searching for, in the worst case, is in the order of minutes. To perform the timestamp synchronization we implement the following steps (Fig. 5).

1. We record a first video i during which we perform a *synchronization event*.
2. We select the event starting frame F_i^{event} from the video and encode it in timestamp format in milliseconds T_i^{event}.
3. We select from the sensors raw data a data time window of 4 min W_i^{sync}, where T_i^{event} refers to the middle point of the window. Within this time window we search for the synchronization event.
4. We identify the event starting time in milliseconds T_i^{sync} within the W_i^{sync}, and we calculate the synchronization time shift $S^i = |T_i^{sync} - T_i^{event}|$, which subsequently is applied to all the data collected during session i.

This procedure has a sort of analogy to the audio-video synchronization procedure in a film production. Also in that case, audio and video signals are recorder independently. In order to synchronize the two, the producer creates a characteristic event using a clapperboard which can be recognized in both audio and video signals.

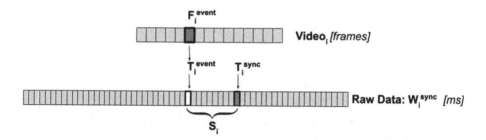

Fig. 5. First step synchronization

4.2   Identification of the Synchronization Event

In order to generate the synchronization event, we performed a characteristic movement with the toy (the reference toy for this analysis is a *cube*). In particular we overturn the toy to stand on a different face, multiple times (minimum 2 times). We exploited also different movements (i.e., trowing the toy, lifting and spinning the toy), resulting in a lower accuracy synchronization. The reference signal we exploit for synchronization is the acceleration, and in particular we implemented the T_i^{sync}-search procedure on the acceleration axis over which the toy is overturned.

Considering the data recorded during the synchronization overturning movement: the data are first filtered for removing the signal noise; subsequently the derivative of the signal is calculated and exploited for the event identification.

In order to use the acceleration data collected while performing the synchronization event to identify the T_i^{sync} we process the signal through a low pass filter for signal noise removal: we decided to use a filter which works on the spatial domain (a Gaussian filter), instead of a frequency domain filter which might add some signal artifacts. In Fig. 6 the row signal is represented in blue, the filtered signal without noise is in orange. Afterwards we calculate a discrete derivative on the filtered signal, in order to detect the time of the synchronization event (green in Fig. 6).

The derivative values have a normal distribution with zero mean. We then identify the synchronization time, the first time the derivative signal values falls outside the interval $[\mu - 1.45 * \sigma, \mu + 1.45 * \sigma]$ (where $\mu = 0$ and σ are mean and standard deviation of the derivative signal). The 1.45 multiplicative factor has been chosen empirically. The result is depicted in Fig. 6, where the red line is a step function, different from zero when the toy is performing an overturn movement, and the vertical solid yellow line corresponds to the identified T_i^{sync}.

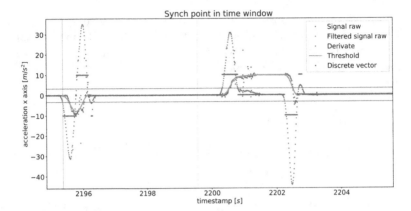

Fig. 6. Acceleration data: example of synchronization procedure with four overturn movements (Color figure online)

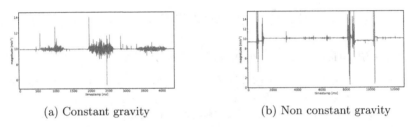

(a) Constant gravity   (b) Non constant gravity

Fig. 7. Measured acceleration magnitude

At this point we can calculate the synchronization time shift as reported in Eq. 1.

$$S^i = \left| T_i^{sync} - T_i^{event} \right| \tag{1}$$

4.3   Gravity Acceleration Removal

As part of the data preprocessing, we had to discriminate signal noise (*non-activity*) from actual toy movement (*activity*), this allows the second step of the synchronization: post-synchronization data-time alignment.

In order to be able to differentiate between activity and non-activity we need to first remove the constant gravitational component from the acceleration data. For this task we work on the *magnitude* of the acceleration vector.

The acceleration magnitude signal is the sum of two components: a dynamic component, proportional to the sum of the forces applied to the sensor node, and a constant component, which correspond to the gravity. In our case, the collected signal, besides being very noisy, it does not always have a longitudinally constant gravity component, however it can change over time. This clearly adds complexity to the synchronization task. For the case of a sampled signal with constant gravity (see Fig. 7a), we remove the gravity component with an high pass filter with cut off frequency $f_c = 0.001\,\text{Hz}$. For the case of a sampled signal with non constant gravity (see Fig. 7b), instead, we use a *Notch filter*, with *parameter* $\lambda = 0.7$: the selected value minimizes the effects of the filter due to the applied transfer function. Focusing on the goal of this task, we need to select a filter which removes the gravitational component, producing an output signal which allows us to differentiate activity from non-activity. Applying the Notch filter with the specified parameter value, produces some changes to the original signal but has a faster response in the gravity removal task, compared to other filters and parameter values.

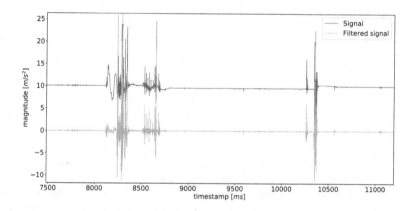

Fig. 8. Example of application of Notch filter, $\lambda = 0.7$ (Color figure online)

Figure 8 represents an example of application of the Notch filter on a non-constant gravity acceleration signal: in blue the magnitude of the acceleration raw data, and in orange the result of the applied filter.

4.4 Activity Discretization: Differentiation Between Activity/Non-activity

In order to finally differentiate between activity and non-activity we perform a statistical analysis of the acceleration signal values. From the acceleration dataset $<a_x, a_y, a_z>$ we compute the features vector $<p_a^n, m_a>$ where:

- p_a^n corresponds to the *power* of the acceleration magnitude $\bar{m}_a$, filtered for gravity removal, calculated over a window of n samples;
- m_a corresponds to the per-sample magnitude of the acceleration, calculated after the application of the gravity removal filter, independently on each axis of the acceleration.

We study the distribution of the computed feature values for two acceleration signals, both corresponding to a time window of 30 s, one referred to an *activity* session (signal generated by the concatenation of different real activity signals), and the other related to a *non-activity* session, both sampled at $100, 21\,\text{Hz}$. For the power feature, we evaluate the impact of the window size (number of samples n) on the values distribution.

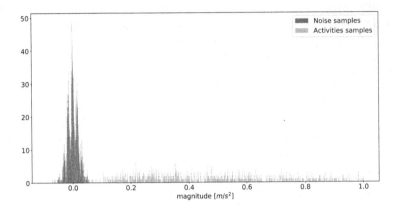

Fig. 9. Magnitude values distribution

Figure 9 represents the distribution of magnitude values m_a for both acceleration signals. While Fig. 10 represents an example of distribution of the power values p_a^8, for an averaging window of 8 samples. For both figures, the blue bars are referred to non-activity signal, while the orange bars are referred to activity.

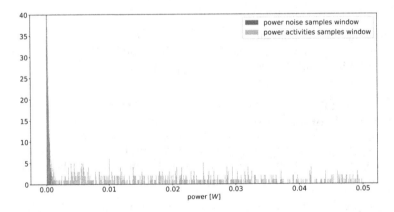

Fig. 10. Power values distribution, dimension of the averaging window $n = 8$

In both cases we can identify a *threshold value* for the data discretization, and for the power feature we can also identify a *window size* value. In order to identify these parameters, we implement an *error minimization* approach, calculating the error in time, over a signal which is associated with its ground truth (start and stop time of each activity). The error is measured in time (milliseconds) as the absolute value of the difference between the ground truth data and the computed signal discretization (activity/non-activity), varying the discretization parameters (threshold and window size).

For the case of signal power based discretization, we applied threshold values in the range of $th_{power} = [0.001; 0.036]$ selected empirically. We applied window size values in the range $n = [2; 18]$. Window size is determined by some domain constraints: the minimum size of an intentional movement of an infant corresponds to 2 video frames (recorded at 25 fps), which means 8 samples of acceleration data (sampled at 100, 21 Hz).

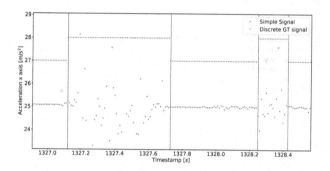

Fig. 11. Single signal with associated GT

Figure 12 shows the sum of absolute error calculated over a single signal (Fig. 11) involving four changes of state (activity/non-activity). We can see from the graph that a window of size $n = 7$ (approximately the length of two video frames) reached a minimum error with threshold values in the range $th_{power} = [0.008; 0.036]$.

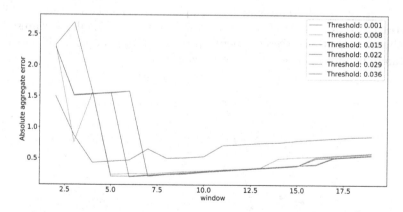

Fig. 12. Sum of absolute error calculated over a single signal, discretization on signal power

In order to implement a more accurate solution, we perform the signal discretization over a multiple sources signal. The assumption for this solution is that all involved sources (sensor nodes) are synchronized with each other. In this case we perform an *Aggregate Error Minimization*: the error minimization task is applied to all the sensors data, computing an *aggregate sum of absolute error*.

This results in a convergence curve: the aggregated error converges to a value. The search for the convergence value stops when the procedure calculates 5 consecutive equal error values. Figure 13 represents the convergence curve of the aggregated error calculated over a real experiment. In this case, for all window sizes $n = [8; 12]$, the convergence value for an optimal aggregate error corresponds to a threshold of $th_{power} = 0.015$.

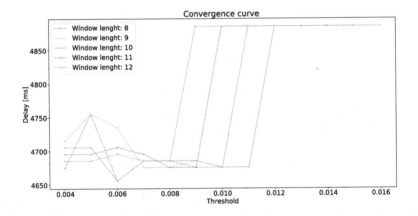

Fig. 13. Convergence curve

We performed a qualitative evaluation of the discretization procedure on the sampled data. Figure 14 represents an example of optimal delays found at different threshold values, with a fixed window size of $n = 10$. The delay represented in the figure is the time difference between the GT timestamp and the raw data timestamp, before the first step synchronization.

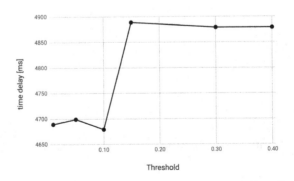

Fig. 14. Delay vs threshold on power discretization, window size $n = 10$

This discretization procedure can be seen as a binary classification task, where the positive class is the *activity* and the negative class in the *non-activity*. Lowering the threshold value we increase the True Positives (activity correctly identified as activity), however very low threshold values increases the False Positives (real non-activity, as signal noise, identified as activity). Increasing the threshold value we increase the False Negatives (real activity identified as non-activity).

Figure 15 represents an example of the discretization procedure on the sampled data. All the lines are step functions equal to 0 in correspondence of *non-activity*, and 1 for the *activity* (the signals have been translated vertically for visualization purposes). The blu plot represents the aggregated ground truth (aggregated over multiple sensors) and generated from the video recording: the signal is equal to 1 if, from the recorded video, the infant is performing a manipulation activity with one of the available toys. The orange plot represents the same signal plotted above after the application of the overall synchronization time shift. The green plot is referred to the acceleration data: it is the result of the discretization procedure based on power feature, with parameter values $th_{power} = 0.030, n = 10$. Analogue results are reached with all the rest of the data in the sample dataset.

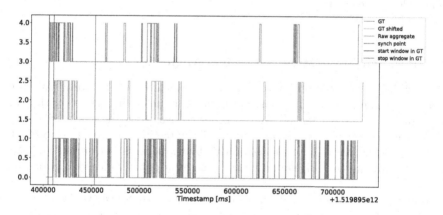

Fig. 15. Discretization example, $th = 0.030, n = 10$

We can see in Fig. 16 the application of both the discratization procedure based on power and on magnitude. The procedure has been applied to a single sensor data for visualization purposes. In the figure, the blue plot represents the sampled acceleration magnitude, while the green data corresponds to the acceleration magnitude after removing the gravitational component. All the remaining signals have been translated vertically for visualization purposes (for all of them, the real minimum value is 0). In brown the result of the discretization based on power (power in orange). In pink the result of the discretization based on magnitude (magnitude in grey). In red the infant activities identified in the ground truth video recordings. Both methods perform well, however in the case of magnitude based approach the results present an higher value of False Positives (real non-activity identified as activity). We decide then to implement the power based method.

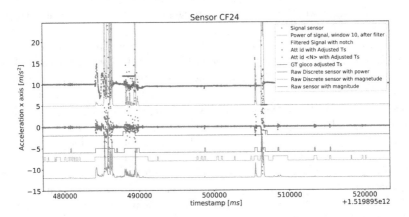

Fig. 16. Discretization procedure application on a single sensor signal raw acceleration data (Color figure online)

4.5   Post-synchronization Data Time Alignment

We described above the procedure for the identification of the overall synchronization time shift between sensors data and video recording. However the synchronization requires a second step in order to deal with the clock drift issue: each measurement session requires a specific data-time alignment in order to adjust the synchronization error introduced by the sensors clock drift. This step is also required in the BLE measurement configuration, introduced in paragraph Sect. 3.

When we perform the *post-synchronization data alignment* we have to consider two important issues. One consists in the fact that we have a video recorded ground truth sampled at a frequency of $f_{video} = 25$ Hz, while the IMU data is sampled at $f_{data} = 100.21$ Hz ($f_{data} = 504.12$ Hz for the car). When we perform the alignment of the ground truth with the raw data, we have to consider the fact that the two frequencies are not multiples of each other. A second issue is related to the information present in the GT data, and in the collected raw data: the reference GT associated to a video consists in a list of all the activities performed by the child, with related information about first and last frame of the activity; the raw data instead includes information about all the movements of the toy, including the movements not directly related to the activities of the infant (e.g., interaction with the educator, with other toys, with the surrounding environment). The usage of the aggregated raw data (data collected by more than one sensor) reduces the effects of this last issue. These issues however force a lower bound for the data synchronization error: the acceptable error is in the range $[-40, +40]$ ms, where 40 ms corresponds to the interval of time between two video frames, and 10 ms corresponds to the interval of time between two inertial sample data.

In order to apply the post-synchronization alignment, we perform a similarity analysis between the *synchronized aggregated raw data discretization signal* and the related *aggregated GT discretization signal*. This analysis has the goal to maximize the similarity between the two signals, searching for the maximum similarity when performing a convolution of a portion of the *GT signal* (typically one half of the GT time series) over the one related to raw data. This procedure allows the identification of a *per-measurement time alignment* which is then applied to the data, as a final step of the synchronization and data pre-processing procedure.

4.6   Final Results

Summarizing the analysis described above, in order to align the raw sensor data to the GT signal we apply a time shift correction to the raw sensor data, as reported in Eq. 2: where j refers to a measurement session recording, while i refers to a prior synchronization event video. Equation 3 represents the delay component $D_{i,j}$, which corresponds to the sum of two time intervals. dt_i^{sync} is the delay measured during the first synchronization phase, while dt_j^{align} is the time alignment delay for the specific measurement j.

$$T_{i,j}^{data} + D_{i,j} = T_j^{video} \tag{2}$$

$$D_{i,j} = dt_i^{sync} + dt_j^{align} \tag{3}$$

As a result of the analysis described in this work, we have a data-set of sensor data with associated GT, ready for the application of machine learning algorithms for infant ludic behavioural analysis.

5   Conclusions and Future Works

5.1   Conclusions

We presented in this work a sensor data-driven synchronization methodology and its application within a multi-sensor environment, storing different types of data (inertial data and video recordings) at different sampling frequencies. In order to apply the presented methodology, network communication between the devices is not required. The presented methodology consists in a two steps procedure: the first one performs the synchronization between the sensor nodes data and the recorded videos; while the second step synchronization allows the data-time alignment when a sensor data clock drift is present. The methodology has been implemented within the context of the AutoPlay project, involving infants and toys for the data acquisition, in a constrained environment.

5.2   Future Works

The proposed procedure works well in the test pilot environment. However, we are currently working on future developments. In the current state of the work, we do not include the ball in the synchronization procedure, for which we are developing a different procedure for generating a reliable synchronization event. Moreover, we are implementing a machine learning algorithm for the signal discretization: building a binary classifier in order to recognize if a given signal refers to a toy manipulation activity or not.

Acknowledgment. This work was supported by Gebert Rüf Stiftung (GRS-054/16). We thank SUPSInido and CullaBabyStar for their support and involvement during the measurement pilot study. We would also like to show our gratitude to all the families which contributed to the project, allowing their kids to participate to the pilot study. Additionally we thanks all SUPSI students and collaborators which have been involved during the GT logs generation, and during the pilot study for the sensor devices and the measuring environments management.

References

1. Bennett, T.R., Gans, N., Jafari, R.: Data-driven synchronization for internet-of-things systems. ACM Trans. Embed. Comput. Syst. **16**(3), 69:1–69:24 (2017). https://doi.org/10.1145/2983627
2. Elson, J., Girod, L., Estrin, D.: Fine-grained network time synchronization using reference broadcasts. ACM SIGOPS Oper. Syst. Rev. **36**(SI), 147–163 (2002)
3. Faraci, F.D., et al.: Autoplay: a smart toys-kit for an objective analysis of children ludic behavior and development. In: 2018 IEEE International Symposium on Medical Measurements and Applications (MeMeA), pp. 1–6. IEEE (2018)
4. Ganeriwal, S., Kumar, R., Srivastava, M.B.: Timing-sync protocol for sensor networks. In: Proceedings of the 1st International Conference on Embedded Networked Sensor Systems, pp. 138–149. ACM (2003)
5. Guidoni, D.L., Boukerche, A., Oliveira, H.A., Mini, R.A., Loureiro, A.A.: A small world model to improve synchronization algorithms for wireless sensor networks. In: The IEEE symposium on Computers and Communications, pp. 229–234. IEEE (2010)
6. Harashima, M., Yasuda, H., Hasegawa, M.: Synchronization of wireless sensor networks using natural environmental signals based on noise-induced phase synchronization phenomenon. In: 2012 IEEE 75th Vehicular Technology Conference (VTC Spring), pp. 1–5. IEEE (2012)
7. Huang, Y.H., Wu, S.H.: Time synchronization protocol for small-scale wireless sensor networks. In: 2010 IEEE Wireless Communication and Networking Conference, pp. 1–5. IEEE (2010)
8. Jain, S., Sharma, Y.: Optimal performance reference broadcast synchronization (OPRBS) for time synchronization in wireless sensor networks. In: 2011 International Conference on Computer, Communication and Electrical Technology (ICCCET), pp. 171–175. IEEE (2011)
9. Lukac, M., Davis, P., Clayton, R., Estrin, D.: Recovering temporal integrity with data driven time synchronization. In: Proceedings of the 2009 International Conference on Information Processing in Sensor Networks, pp. 61–72. IEEE Computer Society (2009)

10. Qiu, T., Liu, X., Han, M., Li, M., Zhang, Y.: SRTS: a self-recoverable time synchronization for sensor networks of healthcare IoT. Comput. Netw. **129**, 481–492 (2017)
11. Skiadopoulos, K., et al.: Synchronization of data measurements in wireless sensor networks for IoT applications. Ad Hoc Netw. **89**, 47–57 (2019)
12. Yildirim, K.S., Kantarci, A.: Time synchronization based on slow-flooding in wireless sensor networks. IEEE Trans. Parallel Distrib. Syst. **25**(1), 244–253 (2013)

A Real-Time Algorithm for PPG Signal Processing During Intense Physical Activity

Andrea Gentili[1(✉)], Alberto Belli[1], Lorenzo Palma[1], Salih Murat Egi[2], and Paola Pierleoni[1]

[1] Department of Information Engineering (DII), Università Politecnica delle Marche, Via Brecce Bianche 12, 60131 Ancona, Italy
a.gentili@pm.univpm.it
[2] Department of Computer Engineering, Galatasaray University, Istanbul, Turkey

Abstract. Photopletismography (PPG) is a simple, low cost and non-invasive technique, implemented by pulse-oximeters to measures several clinical parameters, such as hearth rate, oxygen saturation (Spo$_2$), respiration and other clinical diseases. Although monitoring of these parameters at rest does not present particular problems, processing PPG signals during intensive physical activity is still a challenge, due to the presence of motion artifacts that affect its true estimation. In our work, a novel time-frequency based algorithm is presented to properly reconstruct PPG signal during intensive physical activity with respect to the ECG signal reference. Starting from raw PPG and acceleration signals, the proposed algorithm initially removes motion artifacts, providing an accurate heart rate estimation. Subsequently, it reconstructs PPG waveform based on both the heart rate information previously computed and the optimal selection of frequency-domain components representing PPG signal. Evaluating our proposed method on a dataset containing signals acquired during high speed running, we found for heart rate estimation an average absolute error of 1.20 BPM and very similar frequency dynamics between the ECG reference and PPG reconstructed HRV time series from a physiological point of view based on visual inspection.

Keywords: PPG monitoring · HR estimation · Motion artifacts

1 Introduction

Photopletismography (PPG) is a simple, low cost and noninvasive technique, implemented by pulse-oximeters, aimed to measures various clinical parameters, such as hearth rate (HR), oxygen saturation (Spo$_2$), respiration and other clinical diseases [2]. A pulse oximeter is a small and inexpensive device that measures the changes in arterial blood volume during the cardiac cycle, through the measurement of light-absorption increase due to the systolic increase in arterial blood volume for HbO_2 and Hb, generally in the red and infrared regions [9]. PPG signal may be recorded from fingertip, ear, forehead or wrist. Thus, it is popular in wearable devices such as smart watches or wristbands to measure heart rate in real time [16] also allowing remote monitoring of physiological parameters through web technologies [12]. There are many promising applications for PPG monitoring, although currently they are mainly used on patients at rest, because PPG signal acquired, especially from wrist, is vulnerable to motion artifact (MA) [7]. The amount of MA added depends on the type of physical exercise and hand movement, or many other anomalies, including shifts in light coupling between tissue and sensor, mechanical pulsation of arterial blood irregular with true pulse rate and increase in sensor touch pressure. Thus, MA contamination on PPG signal result in unreliable Spo_2 and HR estimation, making this last a challenge. Developing a robust HR estimation algorithm for wearable devices capable of properly estimating HR in the presence of severe MA is therefore a challenge, as the common filtering method does not remove MA noise as the frequency spectrum of this noise overlaps with that of the true PPG signal. Several techniques for MA detection and removal have been proposed in the literature. Some methods rely on adaptive filtering that manages accelerometer data for MA removal. In particular, the spectrum-subtraction-based MA reduction technique [3] removes the acceleration data from that of a PPG signal. The application of adaptive noise cancellation (ANC) [13,19] is a popular technique used to estimate signals corrupted by additional noise or interference, such as MA. The adaptive filter is inherently self-designed through the use of a recursive algorithm that updates the filter parameters. This approach can be used to obtain the desired level of noise rejection, without a prior estimates of the signal or noise. This method requires two inputs: one PPG signal with a distorted signal and a reference noise signal (RNS) with some possible noise correlation to the first source; the latter obtained as a reference input through an acceleration sensor. It is an advantage to use adaptive method for their fast response time and the capability of continuous processing in time-varying conditions. Experimental results showed that this device produced more reliable signals that were stable against motion artifact corruption under typical types of movement, such as the swinging of the arms [10], making this technique probably one of the best candidate for subjects running or walking in the treadmill, other than underwater applications, as HR and Spo_2 monitoring of dives or subjects during water walking or jogging. Moreover, from the literature, there are not many techniques aimed to compute PPG signal reconstruction and heart rate variability analysis, in presence of high motion artifacts. In this paper, a real-time algorithm based on time-frequency domain is presented to estimate HR and properly reconstruct PPG signal. In order to test the validity of the proposed algorithms, tests were performed on standard signals available in the literature.

2 Methods and Materials

The PPG signals acquired from wrist under intense physical activity has several drawbacks such as poor signal quality and MA corruption. We propose an algorithm that is able to overcome this issue even in the worst conditions. While poor signal quality may be reduced adopting a good pulse oximeter and an suitable filtering method, MA are more difficult to remove. There are mainly three kind of PPG signals, as explained in [1], namely good, bad and worse PPG signal. The first one presents in the spectrum only one peak that represents the true hearth rate. However, this type of PPG signal is not as common when under intense physical exercise as a bad PPG signal. This last contains more than one dominant peak related to true heart rate and MA and its harmonic. Only with an appropriate tracking algorithm can true HR be detected from this type of PPG signal by removing MA. Ultimately, estimating heart rate can be daunting for the worst PPG signal where MA's harmonic peak position is very close to real HR. Availability of these different kind of PPG signals represents a critical aspects in algorithms development for MA reduction. Therefore in this work it is decided to use an online dataset representative of the various case studies. The dataset used in this study [21] is the most used from literature for testing and developing HR estimation algorithms from PPG signals in presence of motion artifacts [11]. The data recorded in the dataset contains two-channel PPG signals and acceleration signals, other than a one-channel ECG signal, recorded simultaneously from subjects, all sampled at 125 Hz. For each subject, the PPG signals were acquired from wrist by two pulse oximeters with the same green LEDs ($\lambda = 609$ nm), whose mutual distance is 2 cm, while the acceleration signals were acquired from a three-axis accelerometer. Both of them are embedded in a wrist-band. The ECG signal was recorded at the same time from the chest of each subject using an ECG sensor. Ground truth values of HR are also available, as reference HR, for comparison in this study. The data of the dataset were acquired from 12 healthy male subjects of age 18–35 years. During the registration process, the subjects walked or ran on a treadmill with a variable speed ranging from 6–8 km/h to 12–15 km/h, each data with an approximate duration of 5 min. The provided dataset was used according to the following ground rules for the detection of heart rate from the PPG signal. The heart rate must be calculated from a time window of eight seconds overlapping six seconds from the previous window, also using the previous data up to the current window, but no operations such as moving average filtering or modifying past heart rate estimates based on the current HR estimate.

3   Algorithm Development and Real-Time Implementation

The main purpose of the present work is the development of an algorithm able to properly reconstruct the PPG signal acquired during intense physical activity. A simple figure to illustrate the whole idea of this paper is shown in Fig. 1. This can only be achieved if an accurate heart rate estimation is available. Therefore, the proposed algorithm is composed of two main parts. The first part regards the estimate of the heart rate while the second part concerns the reconstruction of the PPG signal.

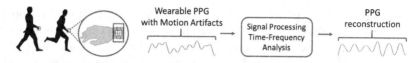

Fig. 1. Simply figure of the proposed algorithm general framework.

3.1   HR Estimation

In this work the estimation of the HR is obtained by processing of raw PPG signals (p_i) and the accelerometer data $(a_j(n))$. $a_j(n)$ denotes motion signals recorded from the three-axis accelerometer sensor, where $n = 0, 1, 2, ...$ denotes sample index and $j = x, y, z$ represents axis index. p_i can be described with a mathematical formulation [15,18], and modelled as:

$$p_i(n) = d_i(n) + w_i(n) \tag{1}$$

where $n = 0, 1, 2, ...$ denotes sample index, $i = 1, 2$ denotes PPG signal index, d_i and w_i represent motion free PPG signal and MA signal, respectively.

In order to estimate the heart rate, we perform a band pass filtering operation on PPG and acceleration data aimed to reduce the random noise introduced due to the sensor probing during recording. A robust HR estimation, during motion, using a recursive least-squares (RLS)-based adaptive filtering technique filters [19,20] and the Sum Slope Function (SSF) [14] with an adaptive threshold scheme from the literature [4]. Finally, we apply a simple peak verification technique to compute the appropriate HR to deal with unexpected estimation of HR. A block diagram of the steps carried out to estimate HR from motion-corrupted PPG signals is shown in Fig. 2 and described in the following.

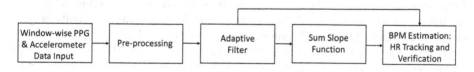

Fig. 2. Block diagram of the proposed method.

Pre-processing. In order to remove noise corresponding to the frequencies outside the range of interest [21], a bandpass filter for pulse detection, of band limits 0.4 Hz to 3.5 Hz, on the two PPG signals and three acceleration signals is applied. Subsequently, an energy normalization and average on the two PPG signals to suppress unwanted random noises [17] is applied. Finally, the two raw PPG recorded signals are averaged, clearly showing more reliability detection of the true heart rate position in its spectrum [1].

Adaptive Filter. After pre-processing, among with several algorithm proposed in the literature, in order to remove MA still present on PPG signal, we adopted adaptive noise cancellation, that need in input both the PPG signal and a reference noise signal, in our case MA. In [1], studying the relationship between MA and acceleration signals, was shown that the dominant peaks of each channel spectrum clearly represent the MA peak in PPG signal spectrum, unlike the spectrum of vector sum of the three accelerometer axes. Thus, in general, taking any one of the acceleration signals as MA noise reference works well in the most of the cases (see Fig. 3). Passing each one, however, as a MA reference, requires more hardware resources and computational power in separate RLS filters.

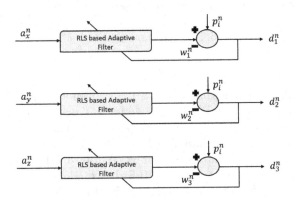

Fig. 3. Block diagram of the RLS-based MA reduction scheme, respectively, for the three accelerometric signals a_x, a_y, a_z.

In this work, we adopted an energy-selective MA reference signal generation from acceleration signals [1]. It is empirically observed that the acceleration signal having greater power band, P_{band}, at specific frequency range, usually in the range of 0.5 Hz to 2 Hz, clearly maintains the maximum dominant peaks correlated with the MA peaks in the PPG spectrum. Therefore, the highest power band acceleration signal is chosen as the MA reference signal. To give the best results, the length of the RLS filter is empirically set to 32. The inverse of covariance matrix is initialized as $10I$, where I is identity matrix of order of RLS filter length. Weight vector is initialized to zero. The RLS forgotten factor is set as 0.999. We have experienced that none of these MA three-axis accelerometers reference signals, taken separately, result in accurate enough estimation of HR for each window, where also the combined RNS vector sum of the three acceleremeter axes fails in most of the cases too. On the other hand, we empirically observed that sometimes, above all on the first two windows, when the subject is considered almost at rest, in presence of a high random noise, the estimation of HR from periodogram is not accurate. At the same time, trying to reduce MA on PPG signal using only one single RLS filtering stage often fails. Thus, only for the first two windows, a second stage with another RNS is implemented, in cascade to the first one, improving the signal to noise ratio (N/R) and the accuracy of the HR estimated, only if the difference between the value of the maxima and the second largest P_{band} is less then 10%. In addition, as some of the windows are so corrupted with MA that only RLS filter doesn't remove the MA correctly, we adopted a further verification step to track the heart rate in the consecutive PPG windows.

Sum Slope Function Algorithm. Heart rate tracking is another key aspect of the proposed method. It results from observation that because the subject on the first two windows is considered at rest, the pulse peaks, in several cases, could be more accurately detected in the time-domain than a spectral tracking, in which the presence of a low signal to noise ratio (S/N) due to random noise can make the HR estimation inaccurate. We chosen to use the Sum Slope Function (SSF) and a peaks finding with adaptive threshold scheme technique [4]. In addition, SSF improves PPG waveform recovery and suppresses the rest of the waveform [22]. The SSF, at time i, SSF_i is defined as:

$$SSF_i = \sum_{k=i-w}^{i} \Delta x_k \ where \ \Delta x_k = \begin{cases} \Delta s_k : \Delta s_k > 0 \\ 0 : \quad \Delta s_k \leq 0 \end{cases} \qquad (2)$$

where w and s_k are the length of the analyzing window and the filtered PPG signal, respectively. In this study, is used the analyzing window size of 0.128 ms for the sampling rate of 125 Hz. Generally, the SSF onset completely coincides with the pulse onset and the pulse peak is totally appeared in the range between the SSF onset and the SSF offset. The algorithm then locates the SSF onset and the SSF offset first and eventually determines the pulse peak within the range as the local limit. Then an adaptive threshold with the SSF and a simple signal conditioning scheme are used to set a search interval for subsequent pulse peak detection by choosing the maximum peak within the search range for a more reliable pulse peak detection. Lastly, overdetected and skipped pulse peaks are deleted and reassessed using knowledge-based rules [6].

Heart Rate Tracking and Verification. Thus, for the first two windows, we used both the SSF and RLS method to better estimate the current HR peak. For the other windows, the heart rate is computed only based on spectral analysis of both RLS filtered PPG and pre-processed PPG signal.

1. HR Estimation for Initial Windows: it is necessary pay a particular attention in the measurement of the first HR windows, because the peaks tracking of the next windows depends on the accuracy of the initial estimate, thus accurate estimation in this step improves the subsequent results. For the first window, if the difference between the current estimated HR with both RLS and SSF method is lower than a fixed value, chosen as 4, $(BPM_{est(SSF)} - BPM_{est(RLS)} < 4)$, the HR of the current window, BPM_{est}, is computed as the average of the two above ($BPM_{est} = 0.50BPM_{est(SSF)} +$

$0.50BPM_{\text{est(RLS)}}$). Otherwise, if the P_{band} of the reference MA acceleration signal is lower than a fixed threshold, P_{th}, ($P_{\text{band}} < P_{\text{th}}$), empirically chosen below which the PPG signal is considered free from MA, the HR of the current window is computed by taking the highest dominant peak location in the RLS-processed PPG signal spectrum ($BPM_{\text{est}} = BPM_{\text{est(RLS)}}$), otherwise, taking that estimated with SSF method ($BPM_{\text{est}} = BPM_{\text{est(SSF)}}$). For the second window, if the difference between the estimated HR with both RLS and SSF method is lower than a fixed value, chosen as 4, ($BPM_{\text{est(SSF)}} - BPM_{\text{est(RLS)}} < 4$), the HR of the current window is computed as the average of the estimated HR with both RLS and SSF method, as above. Otherwise, it simply retain the previous estimate for the current window.

2. Peaks Selection: for the other windows, the current HR is computed, in the most of the windows, finding the maxima dominant peak and the associated location in RLS filtered PPG spectrum. However, may occur cases in which RLS fails to remove MA from PPG signal, because MA is too dominant in the PPG or MA peaks position are too close to heart rate peak location to distinguish them. For this purpose, we set a restricted search range for the current HR peak location, reduced to a specific interval, because the differences between hearts rates of consecutive time windows remains within a small range (due to the biological nature of the signal and the overlapping nature of the windows). Hence, the search interval, for the maximum value dominant peak, was set experimentally as $[R_0 = f_0 - \Delta_R, \ldots, f_0 + \Delta_R]$, where f_0 is the peak location of the estimated HR of the previous window. From this search range, the highest dominant frequency location is obtained, f_{curr} and from which BPM is computed as:

$$\widehat{BPM}_{\text{est}} = \frac{f_{\text{curr}} - 1}{N_{\text{FFT}}} \times 60 \times Fs \tag{3}$$

where Δ_s is set to 6. N_{FFT} is the number of FFT points used for computing spectrum, set to 3000, and F_s is the sampling frequency. Next, a second check is needed on the current estimated peak position, before continuing to further verification steps. Only if the distance between the estimated current HR value, from the maxima dominant peak on the pre-processed PPG signal, $BPM_{\text{pre-processed}}$, and the previously estimated one, $BPM_{\text{est(prev)}}$, is less than the distance between the current HR identified from the RLS filtered PPG signal, $\widehat{BPM}_{\text{est}}$, and that previously estimated, and the corresponding frequency peak in the pre-processed PPG signal spectrum, $f_{\text{pre-processed}}$, is not on reference signal, (f_{acc}, $|(BPM_{\text{pre-processed}} - BPM_{\text{est(prev)}}| < |\widehat{BPM}_{\text{est}} - BPM_{\text{est(prev)}}| \wedge f_{\text{pre-processed}} \neq f_{\text{acc}}$), we took $BPM_{\text{pre-processed}}$ as a value for the current HR peak, ($\widehat{BPM}_{\text{est}} = BPM_{\text{pre-processed}}$).

Otherwise, if the current peak position estimated from the RLS filtered PPG signal is also identified on the reference accelerometric signal and P_{band} of the latter is included in certain values experimentally chosen, P_{th1} and P_{th2} or if the current peak position estimated from the RLS filtered PPG signal do not coincide with that of reference accelerometric signal and the band power of the latter is above the set threshold, P_{th2}, $(f_{cur} \equiv f_{acc} \wedge P_{max} > P_{th1} \wedge P_{max} < P_{th2}) \vee (f_{cur} \neq f_{acc} \wedge (P_{max} > P_{th2})$, the current peak of HR is discarded and taken the second highest peak on the PPG signal periodogram. On the other hand, if the power of the accelerometric reference signal experimentally exceeds another set threshold and the maximum peak position on the pre-processed PPG signal corresponds to that from the RLS filtered PPG signal, then we maintain the valid peak as an estimate of the current HR. So, we take the HR identified as the maximum dominant peak estimated from the RLS filtered PPG signal in all the other cases. This is followed by the verification of the current peak according to the following steps: a smooth heart rate tracking and a verifying procedure in order to prevent extremely high or low estimated values of BPM, to prevent from losing tracking over long time [1].

3.2   PPG Reconstruction

In order to properly reconstruct PPG signal waveform, a promising time-frequency based approach [5] is adopted, from previous literature [5], based on the optimal selection of frequency-domain components that are believe to represent these PPGs, and not include MA. In addition, to improve the accuracy in the PPG signal reconstruction estimation, over each time window, we used our HR information, previously computed. After that, for each time window, we compared the PPG waveform estimated and the position of the associated peaks, with the reference ECG waveform, provided in the dataset.

The previous algorithm is comprised of 5 steps that are illustrated in Fig. 4. A detailed description of these steps are given below in this subsection.

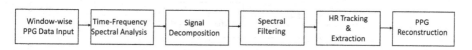

Fig. 4. Block diagram of PPG reconstruction previous algorithm [5].

Time-Frequency Spectral Analysis. The PPG pre-processed signal is down-sampled from the previous frequency of 125 Hz to 20 Hz and the variable frequency complex demodulation (VFCDM) based time-frequency spectrum (TFS) is computed.

Signal Decomposition. The PPG signal is than decomposed into twelve frequency components, according to the frequency bands in the TFS.

Spectral Filtering. Considering HR to be in the range of [0.5 Hz–3 Hz], which typically contains the true HR, considering both low and high pulse rates, is assumed that the largest two peaks and their corresponding frequencies in the PPG spectrum can provide HR information.

HR Tracking and Extraction. If the largest peak is within 10 bpm of the previous HR value, it is chosen; if not, it is checked whether or not the second largest peak is within the 10 bpm range. If the HR value deviates by more than 10 bpm, the HR from the previous window is used.

PPG Reconstruction. The PPG signal is than reconstructed, with the summation of VFCDM components, using only the five components within the anticipated HR range, with frequencies closest to the selected HR during each window. Thus, we used the current BPM_{est}, estimated for each time window, instead of that computed with the previous algorithm, trying to improve the accuracy of the PPG reconstruction (see Fig. 5).

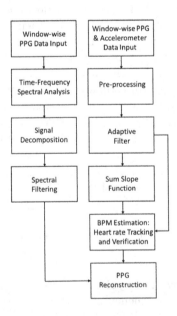

Fig. 5. Block diagram of the proposed PPG reconstruction algorithm.

4   Results

In this work, an algorithm for PPG signal reconstruction was implemented using HR data previously computed for each time window. In order to evaluate the performance of the proposed algorithm for HR estimation, tests were performed on standard signals of dataset available in the literature [21], comprising also an ECG reference signal acquired simultaneously.

The HR estimation results are presented in terms of Average Absolute Error (AAE), defined as:

$$AAE = \frac{1}{N} \sum_{w=1}^{N} |BPM_{\text{est}}(w) - BPM_{\text{true}}(w)| \qquad (4)$$

where BPM_{est} and BPM_{true} are estimated and true value of heart rate in BPM of the w-th window and N is the total number of time windows. The AAE and its standard deviation value (σ) is 1.20 and 1.09, respectively. In Figs. 6 and 7 respectively is shown the best and the worst performing subject, respect to their ground truth values, computed from ECG.

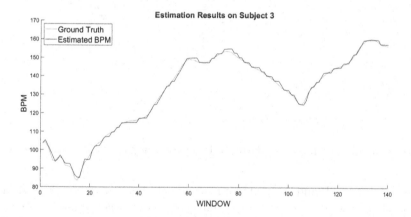

Fig. 6. Performance of the proposed method in subject 3 (best subject).

In order to evaluate the performance of the proposed method for HR estimation, two indices are taken into account, such as Pearson correlation (r) and Bland-Altman plot. Pearson correlation is a measure of degree of similarity between true and estimated values of heart rate. Higher the value of r, better

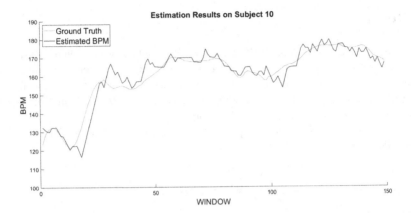

Fig. 7. Performance of the proposed method in subject 10 (worst subject).

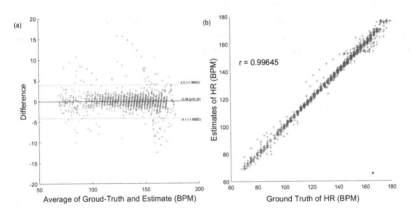

Fig. 8. Estimation results on 12 datasets: Blant-Altman plot (a) Pearson Correlation plot (b).

the estimates. The Bland-Altman plot measures the agreement between true and estimates of heart rate. Here limit of agreement (LOA) is computed using the average difference μ and the standard deviation σ, which is defined as $[\mu - 1.96\sigma, \mu + 1.96\sigma]$. The Pearson correlation coefficient, r, is found 0.9964 and shown in Fig. 8 (left). Next, Blant-Altman plot is shown in Fig. 8 (right), using all time frames of all 12 subjects. The LOA obtained is $[-4.1, 4.0]$.

Both the average absolute error and its standard deviation of HR estimation with our discussed method resulted significantly lower over all 12 subjects (see Table 1). To our knowledge, our algorithm presents very similar accuracy values with respect to the best ones present in the literature, and presenting a lower computational power than most of them.

Table 1. Performance comparison in terms of AEE considering all 12 subjects recording.

Subjects	Previous method	Proposed method
Set. 1	3.65 ± 2.74	1.39 ± 1.67
Set. 2	4.10 ± 2.86	1.28 ± 1.70
Set. 3	4.59 ± 3.31	0.73 ± 0.54
Set. 4	3.78 ± 2.77	1.34 ± 1.67
Set. 5	3.97 ± 2.95	0.82 ± 1.07
Set. 6	3.57 ± 2.41	1.15 ± 1.42
Set. 7	3.70 ± 2.96	0.88 ± 0.99
Set. 8	3.79 ± 2.67	0.86 ± 0.79
Set. 9	4.54 ± 2.82	0.73 ± 0.50
Set. 10	3.43 ± 2.97	3.09 ± 0.50
Set. 11	3.82 ± 2.20	1.42 ± 1.70
Set. 12	4.15 ± 2.90	0.84 ± 0.61
Average $\pm$ sd	3.92 ± 2.80	1.20 ± 1.09

Figure 9(a) shows the comparison between pre-processed and PPG reconstructed signal with our method, while Fig. 9(b) shows a zoomed version of the HRV time series obtained from our and the previous method respectively compared with the reference ECG signal concurrently acquired. Physiologically, PPG signal intensity is maximum at the end of diastole, decreasing during systole, when blood is ejected from the left ventricle into the vascular system, hence increasing the peripheral arterial blood volume, as showed in Fig. 10. Thus, from a qualitative point of view, we are able to estimate quite accurate heart rates and it can be observed similar frequency dynamics between the ECG reference and reconstructed HRV time series with our method, better than those obtained with the previous method.

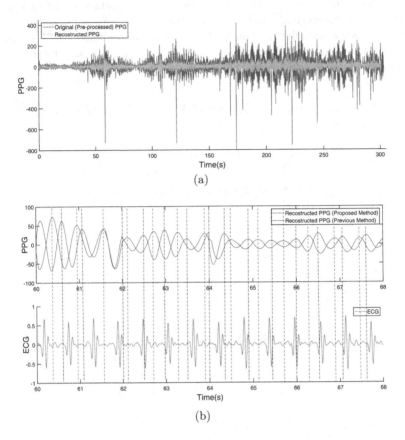

Fig. 9. PPG reconstruction (Dataset 1): (a) previous pre-processed and PPG reconstructed signal with the proposed method from the training dataset, (b) Comparison between PPG signal reconstructed with the proposed method and previous method with reference ECG signal.

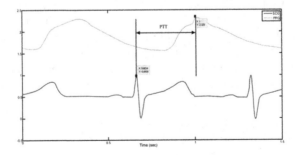

Fig. 10. Pulse transit time (PTT), defined as the time interval between the R-peak of ECG and that of PPG within the same cardiac cycle [8].

5 Conclusions

In this study, we presented a real-time technique based on time-frequency domain to reduce motion artifacts from PPG signals, taken from an online dataset containing MA, in order to reconstruct the associated waveform on 12 subjects data windows during high speed running. From the results obtained, we are able to estimate quite accurate heart rates, observing similar frequency dynamics between the ECG reference and reconstructed HRV time series. The proposed algorithm may have the potential to compute heart rate variability analysis on the results as well as blood pressure estimation as a clinical aid in the study of cardiovascular diseases. Furthermore, the proposed technique for the reduction of motion artifacts, integrated into a healthcare system, may be used to provide continuous health monitoring without interrupting daily life.

Further studies will be conducted subsequently to improve the proposed technique and obtain quantitative results.

References

1. Ahamed, S.T., Islam, M.T.: An efficient method for heart rate monitoring using wrist-type photoplethysmographic signals during intensive physical exercise. In: 2016 5th International Conference on Informatics, Electronics and Vision (ICIEV), pp. 863–868. IEEE (2016)
2. Allen, J.: Photoplethysmography and its application in clinical physiological measurement. Physiol. Meas. **28**(3), R1 (2007)
3. Fukushima, H., Kawanaka, H., Bhuiyan, M.S., Oguri, K.: Estimating heart rate using wrist-type photoplethysmography and acceleration sensor while running. In: 2012 Annual International Conference of the IEEE Engineering in Medicine and Biology Society, pp. 2901–2904. IEEE (2012)
4. Hahn, M.: An adaptive SSF-based pulse peak detection algorithm for heart rate variability analysis in home healthcare environments. In: International Conference on Ubiquitous Healthcare, pp. 70–71 (2010)
5. Harvey, J., Salehizadeh, S.M., Mendelson, Y., Chon, K.H.: Oxima: a frequency-domain approach to address motion artifacts in photoplethysmograms for improved estimation of arterial oxygen saturation and pulse rate. IEEE Trans. Biomed. Eng. **66**(2), 311–318 (2018)
6. Jang, D.G., Farooq, U., Park, S.H., Hahn, M.: A robust method for pulse peak determination in a digital volume pulse waveform with a wandering baseline. IEEE Trans. Biomed. Circuits Syst. **8**(5), 729–737 (2014)
7. Jubran, A.: Pulse oximetry. Crit. Care **3**(2), R11 (1999)
8. Ma, H.T.: A blood pressure monitoring method for stroke management. BioMed Res. Int. **2014**, 1–7 (2014)
9. Nitzan, M., Romem, A., Koppel, R.: Pulse oximetry: fundamentals and technology update. Med. Devices (Auckl. NZ) **7**, 231 (2014)
10. Wei, P.: A new wristband wearable sensor using adaptive reduction filter to reduce motion artifact. In: International Conference on Information Technology and Applications in Biomedicine, ITAB 2008. IEEE (2008)
11. Periyasamy, V., Pramanik, M., Ghosh, P.K.: Review on heart-rate estimation from photoplethysmography and accelerometer signals during physical exercise. J. Indian Inst. Sci. **97**(3), 313–324 (2017)

12. Pierleoni, P., et al.: An innovative webRTC solution for e-health services. In: 2016 IEEE 18th International Conference on E-health Networking, Applications and Services (Healthcom), pp. 1–6. IEEE (2016)
13. Ram, M.R., Madhav, K.V., Krishna, E.H., Komalla, N.R., Reddy, K.A.: A novel approach for motion artifact reduction in PPG signals based on AS-LMS adaptive filter. IEEE Trans. Instrum. Meas. **61**(5), 1445–1457 (2011)
14. Rankawat, S.A., Rankawat, M., Dubey, R.: Heart rate estimation from non-cardiovascular signals using slope sum function and Teager energy. In: 2015 International Conference on Industrial Instrumentation and Control (ICIC), pp. 1534–1539. IEEE (2015)
15. Seyedtabaii, S., Seyedtabaii, L.: Kalman filter based adaptive reduction of motion artifact from photoplethysmographic signal. In: Proceedings of World Academy of Science, Engineering and Technology, vol. 27 (2008)
16. Tamura, T., Maeda, Y., Sekine, M., Yoshida, M.: Wearable photoplethysmographic sensors-past and present. Electronics **3**(2), 282–302 (2014)
17. Temko, A.: Estimation of heart rate from photoplethysmography during physical exercise using Wiener filtering and the phase vocoder. In: 2015 37th Annual International Conference of the IEEE Engineering in Medicine and Biology Society (EMBC), pp. 1500–1503. IEEE (2015)
18. Wood, L.B., Asada, H.H.: Low variance adaptive filter for cancelling motion artifact in wearable photoplethysmogram sensor signals. In: 2007 29th Annual International Conference of the IEEE Engineering in Medicine and Biology Society, pp. 652–655. IEEE (2007)
19. Yousefi, R., Nourani, M., Ostadabbas, S., Panahi, I.: A motion-tolerant adaptive algorithm for wearable photoplethysmographic biosensors. IEEE J. Biomed. Health Inform. **18**(2), 670–681 (2013)
20. Yousefi, R., Nourani, M., Panahi, I.: Adaptive cancellation of motion artifact in wearable biosensors. In: 2012 Annual International Conference of the IEEE Engineering in Medicine and Biology Society, pp. 2004–2008. IEEE (2012)
21. Zhang, Z., Pi, Z., Liu, B.: TROIKA: a general framework for heart rate monitoring using wrist-type photoplethysmographic signals during intensive physical exercise. IEEE Trans. Biomed. Eng. **62**(2), 522–531 (2014)
22. Zong, W., Moody, G., Mark, R.: Reduction of false arterial blood pressure alarms using signal quality assessement and relationships between the electrocardiogram and arterial blood pressure. Med. Biol. Eng. Comput. **42**(5), 698–706 (2004)

Design and Testing of a Textile EMG Sensor for Prosthetic Control

Luisa M. Arruda[1]([✉]) [iD], Alexandre Calado[2] [iD], Rachel S. Boldt[1] [iD],
Yao Yu[1], Helder Carvalho[1] [iD], Miguel A. F. Carvalho[1] [iD],
Fernando B. N. Ferreira[1] [iD], Filomena Soares[2] [iD],
and Demétrio Matos[3] [iD]

[1] Centro de Ciência e Tecnologia Têxtil, University of Minho,
Guimarães, Portugal
luisamendesarruda@gmail.com
[2] Centro Algoritmi, University of Minho, Guimarães, Portugal
[3] Instituto Politécnico do Cávado e do Ave, Barcelos, Portugal

Abstract. Nowadays, Electromyography (EMG) signals generated by the amputee's residual limbs are widely used for the control of myoelectric prostheses, usually with the aid of pattern-recognition algorithms. Since myoelectric prostheses are wearable medical devices, the sensors that integrate them should be appropriate for the users' daily life, meeting the requirements of lightness, flexibility, greater motion identification, and skin adaptability. Therefore, this study aims to design and test an EMG sensor for prosthetic control, focusing on aspects such as adjustability, lightness, precise and constant signal acquisition; and replacing the conventional components of an EMG sensor with textile materials. The proposed sensor was made with *Shieldex Technik-tex P130 + B* conductive knitted fabric, with 99% pure silver plating. EMG data acquisition was performed twice on three volunteers: one with the textile sensor, and other with a commercial sensor used in prosthetic applications. Overall, the textile and the commercial sensor presented total average Signal-to-Noise Ratio (SNR) values of 10.24 ± 5.45 dB and 11.74 ± 8.64 dB, respectively. The authors consider that the obtained results are promising and leave room for further improvements in future work, such as designing strategies to deal with known sources of noise contamination and to increase the adhesion to the skin. In sum, the results presented in this paper indicate that, with the appropriate improvements, the proposed textile sensor may have the potential of being used for myoelectric prosthetic control, which can be a more ergonomic and accessible alternative to the sensors that are currently used for controlling these devices.

Keywords: Textile electrode · EMG · Prostheses

1 Introduction and State-of-the-Art

The scientific community has set goals for advancements in the control of upper limb prosthetic devices, in which specific requirements must be reached: simultaneous, independent, and proportional control of multiple degrees-of-freedom with acceptable

N. M. Garcia et al. (Eds.): HealthyIoT 2019, LNICST 314, pp. 37–51, 2020.

performance and adequate response times [1]. Tom achieve this, intuitive and afford-able methods for better prosthesis control are needed. Due to the simplicity, improvement and affordability of the fused deposition modeling (FDM) 3D printing technique, enabling amputees worldwide to print their upper limb prostheses directly at home, the interest in this subject has been growing immensely [2]. To achieve more responsive and controllable devices, the importance of proper acquisition and pro-cessing of electromyographic (EMG) signals is required. For the success of future prostheses, the sensors that integrate them should be qualified for the daily life of users, meeting the requirements of lightness, flexibility, greater motion identification, long battery life and easy skin adaptability. This study starts from the motivation to develop an ergonomic, viable, flexible sensor that contributes to a more effective and com-fortable control of myoelectric prostheses.

In this sense, although the state of the art has presented the sonomyographic pro-prioceptive method as the most recent non-invasive technique for prosthetic control [3], one of the most used ways to control prosthetic devices is still through the residual limb muscles' EMG signals. This is justified because, although ultrasound allows a more accurate detection of deep muscle compartments in the forearm causing better control compared to traditional myoelectric detection techniques, clinical ultrasound devices, even portable, are too bulky to integrate a prosthetic limb. For this reason, the myo-electric control in this study is the alternative investigated.

In this technique, conductive electrodes detect small electric potentials generated by the exchange of ions through the muscular membranes. The obtained signal is known as myoelectric, and the conversion methodology is called electromyography. Observ-ing these signals and their properties (frequency, amplitude, power and rise time) allows both identifying abnormalities in muscle contraction as well as identifying and classifying different movements performed by the body. More specifically, it is pos-sible to use pattern recognition algorithms to classify the signals obtained by EMG and allow prosthetic devices to recognize such patterns and respond in an expected way [4].

An example of this application is the Myo Armband [5]. Launched commercially in 2013, it is a wearable system for multimedia applications such as games and screen display control that fuses eight channels of EMG sensor information with inertial sensors to achieve gesture recognition. Being a bracelet that is adjustable for various arm dimensions, and that can be positioned in several points to obtain simultaneous signals from distinct forearm muscles, it is suggested as an affordable alternative for myoelectric prosthesis control [6]. There are even prosthetic models available on the internet to be controlled by the Myo armband [7].

With the advent of wearable systems, the interest in using smart textiles in the medical field is intensifying [8, 9]. Textiles are more flexible and adapt better to different designs when compared to conventional electronic structures. Specifically, for prosthesis control, research has been done on textile sensors whose electrodes are composed of conductive inks [10], nickel-plated conductive fabric [11], embroidered electrodes mimicking the archimedean spiral antenna-shaped model, which intends not to establish direct skin contact [12], or even through knitting electrodes made of silver wire [13]. All these studies compare the signals obtained by textile sensors with conventional Ag/AgCl gel electrodes. For instance, in one study knitted textile elec-trodes were used, and the signal to noise-ratio obtained was on average 17.97 dB, better than the 13.3 dB obtained with disposable electrodes [13]. In particular, the antenna model electrode proved that it is capable of detecting signals at a depth of 10 mm, at a distance of 2 and 3 mm application on the skin [12]. Therefore, textile electrodes present several advantages: flexibility, wearability, breathability and easy integration into garments such as sockets used on residual limbs.

The work herein described aims to assess the reliability of one type of construction for textile electrodes, when compared to an EMG sensor already established in the prosthetic market. Furthermore, a comparison of the activation of individual muscles by specific gestures is made, in order to assess the possibility of gesture recognition.

2   Materials and Methods

2.1   Sensor Design

The sensor was designed to fulfill the characteristics of a wearable piece, therefore, the following requirements were listed: adjustability, in order to be adaptable to various body types; lightness, considering that one of the factors of prostheses rejection is the weight of the medical devices [14, 15]; precise and constant signal acquisition, in order to be comparable to sensors already used by the prosthetic market; and replacing the conventional components of a sensor with a textile material, thus bringing it closer to a garment.

The guidelines of the Surface Electromyography (sEMG) for the Non-Invasive Assessment of Muscle Project (SENIAM) were followed [16]. These guidelines are based on recommendations made by countries of the European Union included in the program of Health and Biomedical Research (BIOMED II). The recommendations focus on aspects such as: sensor design (shape, size, distance between electrodes, raw material to use and how to build it); placement of sensors (skin preparation, position and fixation); and location of the muscles for sensor positioning.

To meet the adjustability requirement, the sensor was made of an elastic textile structure, 65% polyester and 35% elastane, with 30 cm of length. A touch fastener with 12 cm was used, which allowed the same sensor to be tested on volunteers whose forearm width ranged from 21 to 30 cm.

Regarding electrode dimensions, the first prototype was composed of circular shaped electrodes, 10 mm in diameter and 20 mm of inter-electrode distance. The material used for the construction of the electrodes was the *Shieldex Technik-tex P130 + B* conductive knitted fabric (78% Polyamide + 22% Elastane), with 99% pure silver plating. The conductive fabric was applied to the aforementioned band with a thermoplastic adhesive (Bemis 5254) at 170° and 5.5 bar for 20 s on the heat press. However, when performing the contact tests whose protocol is described below, only noise was obtained. Therefore, the size of the electrodes was gradually increased, and the shape was changed. The best results were obtained with 2×5 cm rectangular electrodes, using two electrodes and a reference electrode positioned at the most distal part of the forearm (Fig. 1). Thermoplastic polyurethane (TPU) tape and film were used around the electrodes to isolate the detection area for better sensor performance, as previous work has shown [17] (Fig. 2). The textile sensor presented a weight of 17.48 g.

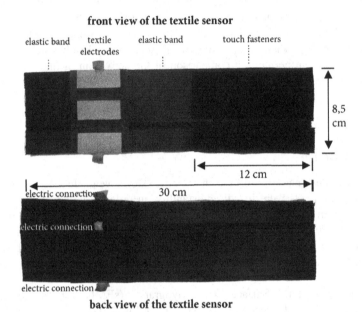

Fig. 1. The figure shows the design and dimensions of the elastic band with the integrated textile electrodes.

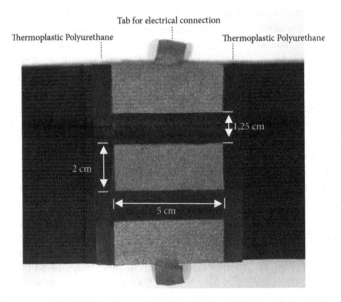

Fig. 2. The figure shows the expanded view of the textile sensor.

In order to have a means of comparison, besides acquiring EMG data with the proposed textile sensor, a commercial sensor was also used. This way, it was possible to grasp a clearer idea of how good the textile sensor performs. For the purposes of this work, an Ottobock 13E68 sensor was used. This sEMG sensor is circular and measures 27.5 mm wide by 13.5 mm high, weighing 9 g, according to the manufacturer (Fig. 3). It is a bipolar model with amplification, internal filtering and enveloping. It is also a sensor used for myoelectric control of prostheses.

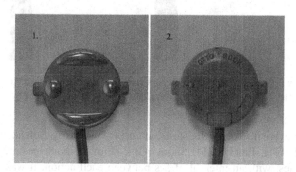

Fig. 3. The figure shows the conventional sEMG model 13E68, manufactured by Ottobock, where 1 is the front view and 2 the back view.

2.2 Subject Information

Three subjects (1 male and 2 female), with 25, 30 and 33 years old, respectively, without any neurological and muscular pathology, were selected to perform the tests. All individuals provided written informed consent and gave permission for the publication of photographs for scientific and educational purposes. The male volunteer will be referred here as V1 and had a 26.5 cm width forearm, volunteer V2 had a 21 cm width forearm, and volunteer V3 had 25 cm width forearm.

2.3 Protocol and EMG Data Acquisition

The EMG data acquisition experiment was performed with each subject. This experiment was composed by two parts. In the first part of the experiment, EMG data was acquired through textile sensors positioned alternately in the *Flexor Carpi Radialis*, *Flexor Carpi Ulnaris*, *Extensor Carpi Ulnaris* and *Extensor Carpi Radialis* muscles. These muscles were selected due to their active contribution to finger and hand movement, as well as their location on the forearm, as they are superficial muscles, which means that the generated signals are easier to detect with surface electromyography (sEMG). In order to identify the location of such muscles in a tactile manner, standard instructions were followed according to the literature [18]. Thereafter, in the second part of the experiment, the Ottobock sensor was positioned at the same locations as the textile sensor (Fig. 4). There was a rest between each test. The time interval between the two parts of the experiment was of one to two days, depending on the availability of volunteers.

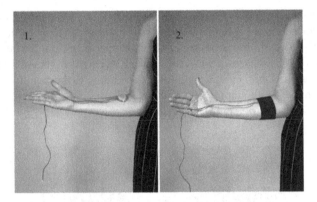

Fig. 4. This image depicts how the commercial sensor (Ottobock) was placed on the volunteers' right forearm with an elastic band similar to the one used with the textile sensor.

Six gestures were listed for the tests, namely: Fist (G1), Spread (G2), Wave-in (G3), Wave-out (G4), Pinch (G5), Shoot (G6), (Fig. 5). Each gesture, in turn, was repeated five times, with an interval of 5 s between each action. It was recommended that the volunteers apply their highest level of isometric force production.

The data acquisition system consisted of a NI USB-6229 data acquisition board with software in LabVIEW. Whilst the signals from the Ottobock sensor were acquired directly, the textile armband was used with the Myoware AT-04-001 muscle sensor for signal conditioning, being its output connected to the data acquisition board. All signals were acquired using a sampling frequency of 1 kHz.

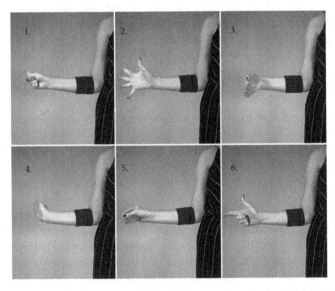

Fig. 5. The image shows the six gestures performed by the volunteers: Fist (G1); Spread (G2); Wave-in (G3); Wave-out (G4); Pinch (G5); Shoot (G6).

2.4   Signal Processing

The sensors manufactured by Ottobock, such as the 13E68, are optimized for prosthetic/myoelectric control purposes, featuring on-board analog amplification, filtering and enveloping, whereas the proposed textile sensor's signal is "raw", i.e. it lacks any signal processing.

All signal processing for the textile sensors was performed digitally in an application developed with LabVIEW. Signals were filtered with a Notch filter at 50 Hz in order to eliminate the power line noise, and a band-pass filter with cut-off frequencies of 10–450 Hz. The latter were chosen considering that the recommended band-pass frequency range is 10–500 Hz [19, 20]. According to the manufacturer's general specifications, Ottobock sensors use a 90 to 450 Hz passband. For the specific sensor used, a notch filter at 50 or 60 Hz is specified [14]. However, it was not possible to confirm the exact specification for the sensor.

The final operation to obtain a smoother and more stable signal is enveloping, which was achieved using a moving average filter. A time window of 300 ms was used, which is appropriate for slow or static activities [20], such as the ones performed during signal acquisition. As previously stated, no signal processing was performed on the EMG signals recorded using the Ottobock sensor.

The quality of the EMG signals was evaluated in terms of the Signal-to-Noise Ratio (SNR), which is a standard method used for this purpose [19]. The SNR can be calculated with Eq. 1, where A_S is the average signal amplitude and A_N is the average noise amplitude.

$$SNR = 20 \log(\frac{A_S}{A_N}) \tag{1}$$

The background noise was considered to the baseline noise and the EMG burst observed while the muscle is contracted is the signal that must be detected.

The SNR was calculated for each recording, which comprised five repetitions of the same gesture (for each sensor position), separated by periods of rest, as described in Sect. 2.3.

To ease the calculation of the SNR, a semi-automatic algorithm for detection of the activation (onset) and idle periods of muscle activity was implemented, based on the double-threshold detection methods suggested in [19]. In this method, the detection of activation depends on the application of an amplitude threshold, as well as a minimum activation time, in order to reject noise spikes and motion artifacts.

Since each recording starts with approximately 5 s of rest, i.e. baseline noise, the baseline was initially defined as the mean voltage of 2 s taken of the initial rest period. The user may then adjust this baseline by dragging the cursor drawn by the software to indicate the baseline.

To compute the amplitude detection threshold, a first attempt was made using the suggested criterion [19] in that the EMG signal must surpass a value that represents the 95% confidence interval ($\mu \pm 1.96\sigma$) for baseline activity. However, this method seemed to define the threshold too low, and even extending to ($\mu \pm 2.58\sigma$) the method revealed not very efficient. It was then decided to calculate the amplitude of the signals and define the threshold as 5% of the amplitude.

The second criterion was to consider a minimum activation time to consider the activation valid. A default value of 2 s was defined.

The automatic detection of the intervals was then graphically represented by cursors. At this moment, it was possible to accept the automatically generated activation/idle intervals, re-generate them with another time threshold, adjust the amplitude threshold manually or adjust the intervals directly, by dragging the cursors.

After this process, SNR was computed based on the generated onsets.

3   Results

Figures 6, 7, 8 and 9 show samples of EMG signals acquired by the Ottobock and textile sensors from the *Extensor Carpi Radialis* muscle in gesture 4, the one that, generally speaking, produced the strongest signals. In this case, the signals belong to subject V1.

The raw signal obtained with the textile sensor is depicted in Figs. 6 and 7 shows the filtered signal, Fig. 8 the envelope computed with the moving average filter. It is also possible to observe the automatically generated baseline, amplitude threshold values, as well as the activation intervals found. The same can be observed in Fig. 9 for the signal of the Ottobock sensor.

It was possible in about 80% of the cases to use the automatically generated values directly, whilst in the remaining cases it was necessary to adjust the parameters and recalculate, or to adjust the intervals explicitly.

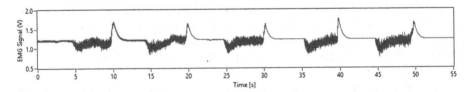

Fig. 6. Raw EMG signal acquired with the textile sensor from subject V1's *Extensor Carpi Radialis* muscle in gesture 4

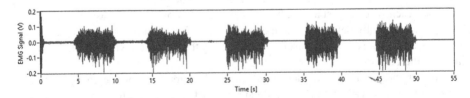

Fig. 7. Bandpass and Notch filtered EMG signal acquired with the textile sensor from subject V1's *Extensor Carpi Radialis* muscle in gesture 4

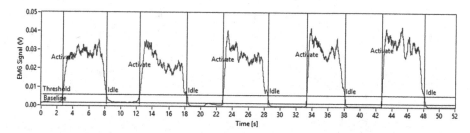

Fig. 8. Enveloped EMG signal acquired with the textile sensor from subject V1's *Extensor Carpi Radialis* muscle in gesture 4. It is also possible observe the automatically generated baseline, amplitude threshold values, and computed activation intervals

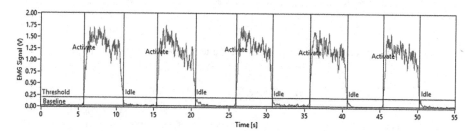

Fig. 9. EMG signal acquired with the Ottobock sensor from subject V1's *Extensor Carpi Radialis* muscle in gesture 4. As in Fig. 8, it is possible observe the automatically generated baseline, amplitude threshold values, and computed activation intervals

Regarding signal acquisition performed with the textile sensor, some issues were observed during two of the sensor positionings, namely for subject V2, in the position above the *Extensor Carpi Radialis*, and for the subject V3, in the position above the *Extensor Carpi Ulnaris*. In both cases, it was not possible to obtain the EMG signal after placing the sensor on the subject's skin surface. This might have occurred due to poor contact between the textile electrode and the skin, or due to some problem regarding the connection between the textile sensor and the EMG MyowareAT-04-001. Regardless, this situation was not verified during the recording performed with the Ottobock sensor. Considering this, the recordings regarding the aforementioned muscles were not considered for the analysis presented in this section.

The results concerning the computation of the SNR are presented in the graphs of Figs. 10 and 11, for the textile and the Ottobock sensor, respectively. The graphs represent the average SNR, in dBs, per sensor position (i.e. per muscle), for each of the three subjects. As previously mentioned in this section, the results regarding the textile sensor positioning on the *Extensor Carpi Radialis* from subject V2 and on the *Extensor Carpi Ulnaris* from subject V3 were not taken into account.

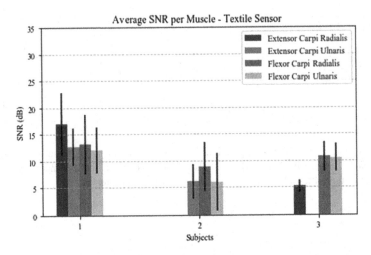

Fig. 10. Average SNR per position for the textile sensor, for each subject

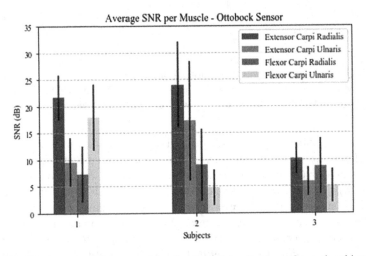

Fig. 11. Average SNR per position for the Ottobock sensor, for each subject

Overall, the total average SNR calculated using the recordings made with the textile sensor was of approximately 10.24 ± 5.45 dB. As for the Ottobock sensor, the total average was of 11.74 ± 8.64 dB.

Taking into account the goal of the present work, it is also relevant to validate, even if only empirically, if the EMG signals acquired with the textile sensor have potential to be used for classification with Machine Learning algorithms, as it is traditionally done in typical myoelectric control systems, such as the ones used in myoelectric transradial prostheses. For this, it is important to check if there are distinct EMG patterns for each of the six gestures. Bearing this in mind, the graph depicted in Fig. 12 represents one muscle activation of the first execution of each gesture, preceded and followed by 2 s of idle time. The plots correspondent to each muscle were artificially synchronized and overlapped in order to simulate the EMG pattern that could be potentially obtained if four textile sensors were being used at the same time. Additionally, the average baseline value was subtracted for each signal, in order to simulate an optimal scenario where the baseline is approximately zero. This was only done for subject V1, as it is the only case where it was possible to acquire signals from all sensor positions with the textile sensor. This type of analysis was not necessary to be performed for the Ottobock sensor's case, as it is a standard sensor used for prosthetic applications.

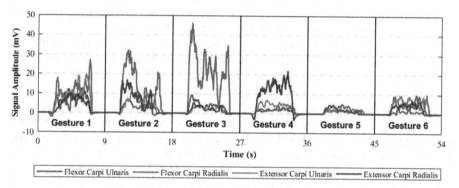

Fig. 12. EMG patterns recorded for each of the six gestures performed by subject V1, taking only into account the first execution of each gesture

4 Discussion

Regarding the results presented in Sect. 3, it is possible to observe in Figs. 10 and 11 that the average SNR varied considerably according to the positioning of both sensors, as well as from subject to subject. These differences might have occurred due to several reasons, such as motion artifacts, of which the main sources are the electrode cable and the electrode interface, as the electrodes can move with respect to each other when the subject performs a gesture [21]. There is also the possibility that the sensors were not placed at the optimal muscle position for all subjects, which could have caused different degrees of crosstalk for each subject, a situation that occurs when an undesired EMG signal generated by a nearby muscle group interferes with the signal generated by the desired muscle. Furthermore, the noise in the EMG signal varies according to the subject's characteristics, such as the tissue structure (which includes muscle and fat), blood flow velocity, skin hair, skin temperature, sweat, among others [22].

A priori, a higher average SNR value (11.74 ± 8.64 dB) was expected for the signals acquired with the Ottobock sensor, as it is already used for prosthetic applications and optimized in terms of materials and signal conditioning. In fact, as observed in Fig. 11, for some sensor positions the average SNR is relatively high, if the results obtained with the textile sensor are taken as comparison. However, for some of the muscle positions, the SNR is also considerably low. This variation in the SNR values is well palpable by considering the high standard deviation (8.64 dB). Besides crosstalk and motion artifacts, the low SNR values for this case could have occurred due to electromagnetic noise, as the human body can behave like an antenna by capturing electric and magnetic radiation from the surrounding environment [22]. It was also possible to observe situations of baseline fluctuation in some of the acquired signals by the Ottobock sensor. This could have happened due the shaking of the electrode cables, as well as electrical drifts in the acquisition equipment [21]. Still regarding the Otto-bock sensor, in other situations the signal was relatively weak and there was difficulty in discerning the periods in which the gesture was being performed. Poor skin-electrode interface could have been the issue in these types of occurrences.

Regardless, the total average SNR of the proposed textile and the Ottobock sensor were similar, although a higher variability of values was observed in the latter. These were positive results, considering that the proposed sensor allowed results comparable to the ones obtained with a commercial sensor. However, the issues encountered during the recording with the Ottobock sensor may have favored the textile sensor on the analysis presented throughout the previous section. Despite this, it is important to take into account the situations previously mentioned regarding the impossibility of acquiring any signal with the textile sensor. Nevertheless, the authors consider that a total average of SNR of 10.24 ± 5.45 dB shows that the obtained results are promising and leave room for further improvements in future work.

Additionally, the obtaining of visibly different EMG patterns for each gesture, as can be observed in Fig. 12, is also a good indicator of the potential of the proposed sensor for classification purposes. For instance, it is interesting to note that the signals corresponding to the sensors placed in the *Extensor Carpi Radialis* and *Extensor Carpi Ulnaris*, which are both muscles responsible for wrist extension, present the highest amplitude values for gesture 4, which is a gesture that includes the extension movement of the wrist. An analogous scenario is also observed between the *Flexor Carpi Radialis* and *Flexor Carpi Ulnaris*, which are responsible for wrist flexion, and gesture 3. Although this is merely an empirical result, it enables the possibility of using an armband with several textile sensors for controlling a multi-degrees-of-freedom prosthesis, which is the main aim of work being developed by the authors. However, due to the reasons stated in the "Results" Section, it is important to bear in mind that the EMG patterns of each gesture were only plotted for one of the subjects. Thus, for now, this type of results cannot be generalized.

5   Conclusions and Future Work

This pilot study proposed to analyze the quality of EMG signals acquired with a textile sensor, in comparison to the quality of the signals acquired with a commercial sensor that is already used in prosthetic control of artificial upper limbs. This analysis was based on the SNR from each recording, which was then averaged per sensor position, for each subject's case, as depicted in Figs. 10 and 11. Overall, the textile and the Ottobock sensor presented total average SNR values of 10.24 ± 5.45 dB and 11.74 ± 8.64 dB, respectively.

Although the average SNR value obtained with the Ottobock sensor was slightly higher, it was expected that it would be even higher, considering the quality of the sensor. In order to tackle the issues encountered with the use of this sensor, more attention should be given to sensor positioning in order to avoid a high degree of crosstalk, as well as ensuring there is an adequate interface between the sensor and the subject. Electromagnetic noise may also be decreased with adapting filtering strategies [22]. Furthermore, baseline fluctuation can also be corrected with a correct fixation of the electrodes [21].

Nonetheless, in comparison with the Ottobock sensor, the results obtained with the textile sensor were considered to be satisfactory and encouraging for the development of future work. Further improvements on the quality of the signals acquired with the proposed sensor can be achieved by designing strategies to deal with known sources of noise contamination. For instance, the selection of an appropriate electrode size and inter-electrode distance may help decrease the influence of crosstalk [21, 22]. Also, although the frequency range typically related with motion artifacts (0–10 Hz) was filtered with the bandpass, it is possible that it could have been one of the sources of noise present in signals. To deal with this, more attention must be given to the design of the electronic circuitry [21]. In order to obtain a detection surface (i.e. electrode-tissue interface area) as good as those present in commercial sensors, the use of a chemical component that can act as an electrolyte has been proposed so that, when combined with the textile electrode, it will be possible to increase the adhesion to the skin.

Another aspect to have into account concerns the impedance of the skin. It is recommended that, for better signal acquisition, impedance should be reduced by removing hair on the skin [23]. However, since a prosthesis is a medical device for daily use, alternatives are needed that minimize impedance without the need to remove them.

It is also important to note that differential amplification and filtering is done on the Ottobock sensor directly, whilst the textile sensor is connected to the signal conditioning circuitry through relatively long wires (about 1 m), which is expected to significantly contribute to noise pick-up.

As it was has previously mentioned, five requirements for the execution of the sensor were listed. Regarding adjustability, the choice of an elastic band with touch fasteners allowed the test to be performed on arms with a variation of up to 10 cm, which proves the contemplation of a diverse audience.

In the lightness category, the manufacturer reports that the Ottobock sensor weights 9 g. On the other hand, the textile sensor weighed 17.48 g. For future projects, such variation may be further reduced or even equated if the amount of touch fasteners is succinct, while maintaining the adjustability feature. Even so, the values are considerable significant for their integration into medical devices.

Regarding the last requirement of the sensor design, that is, the replacement of conventional components by textile materials, the test described in this work showed some lack of constancy of signal acquisition by the developed sensor. It is not yet known whether this factor is exclusively related to the use of a textile-based electrode. Still, since textiles are flexible materials, they become malleable for application in sockets or insertion in any wearable part, that is, they fulfill the comfort requirement for prolonged use of the medical device, besides being lighter than conventional ones.

In sum, the testing of the proposed prototype presented promising results and they indicate that an armband composed by multiple of these sensors can be a more ergonomic and cheaper alternative to the sensors that are currently used for controlling myoelectric prostheses.

Acknowledgments. This work is financed by Project "Deus ex Machina", NORTE-01-0145-FEDER-000026, funded by CCDRN, through Sistema de Apoio à InvestigaçãoCientífica e Tecnológica (Projetos Estruturados I&D&I) of Programa Operacional Regional do Norte, from Portugal 2020 and by Project UID/CTM/00264/2019 of 2C2T – Centro de Ciência e Tecnologia Têxtil, funded by National Founds through FCT/MCTES.

References

1. Jamal, M.Z.: Signal acquisition using surface EMG and circuit design considerations for robotic prosthesis. In: Computational Intelligence in Electromyography Analysis - A Perspective on Current Applications and Future Challengers, pp. 427–445 (2012). https://doi.org/10.5772/52556
2. ten Kate, J., Smit, G., Breedveld, P.: 3D-printed upper limb prostheses: a review. Disabil. Rehabil. Assist. Technol. **12**, 300–314 (2017). https://doi.org/10.1080/17483107.2016.1253117
3. Dhawan, A.S., et al.: Proprioceptive sonomyographic control: a novel method for intuitive and proportional control of multiple degrees-of-freedom for individuals with upper extremity limb loss. Sci. Rep. **9**, 1–15 (2019). https://doi.org/10.1038/s41598-019-45459-7
4. Calado, A., Soares, F., Matos, D.: A review on commercially available anthropomorphic myoelectric prosthetic hands, pattern-recognition-based microcontrollers and sEMG sensors used for prosthetic control. In: IEEE International Conference on Autonomous Robot Systems and Competitions (ICARSC 2019), pp. 1–6 (2019). https://doi.org/10.1109/icarsc.2019.8733629
5. Calado, A.: Comparison between low-cost and high-end sEMG sensors for the control of a transradial myoelectric prosthesis (2017). https://doi.org/10.13140/RG.2.2.18311.04008
6. de Jesus Lima, E., Sanca, A., Arabiam, A.: Development of a 3D printed prosthetic myoelectric hand driven by DC actuators. In: XIII Simpósio Brasileiro de Automação Inteligente. Universidade Federal do Rio Grande do Sul, Porto Alegre (2017)
7. Poparaguai: Myo + Po. https://www.thingiverse.com/thing:2409406?fbclid=IwAR1Z4LENh4qfVhHfjvdL9-3k6und4c6JYU9L5ALTgshrEEy0I8_74eUky2Y. Accessed 18 Oct 2019
8. Pantelopoulos, A., Bourbakis, N.G.: A survey on wearable sensor-based systems for health monitoring and prognosis. IEEE Trans. Syst. Man Cybern. Part C Appl. Rev. **40**, 1–12 (2010). https://doi.org/10.1109/TSMCC.2009.2032660
9. Stoppa, M., Chiolerio, A.: Wearable electronics and smart textiles: a critical review. Sens. (Switz.) **14**, 11957–11992 (2014). https://doi.org/10.3390/s140711957
10. Zhang, H., Tian, L., Zhang, L., Li, G.: Using textile electrode EMG for prosthetic movement identification in transradial amputees. In: 2013 IEEE International Conference on Body Sensor Networks, BSN 2013 (2013). https://doi.org/10.1109/BSN.2013.6575510
11. Li, G., Geng, Y., Tao, D., Zhou, P.: Performance of electromyography recorded using textile electrodes in classifying arm movements. In: Proceedings of the Annual International Conference of the IEEE Engineering in Medicine and Biology Society, EMBS, pp. 4243–4246. IEEE EMBS, Boston (2011). https://doi.org/10.1109/IEMBS.2011.6091053

12. Mangezi, A., Rosendo, A., Howard, M., Stopforth, R.: Embroidered archimedean spiral electrodes for contactless prosthetic control. In: IEEE International Conference on Rehabilitation Robotics, pp. 1343–1348 (2017). https://doi.org/10.1109/ICORR.2017.8009435
13. Lee, S., Kim, M.O., Kang, T., Park, J., Choi, Y.: Knit band sensor for myoelectric control of surface EMG-based prosthetic hand. IEEE Sens. J. **18**, 8578–8586 (2018). https://doi.org/10.1109/JSEN.2018.2865623
14. Biddiss, E., Chau, T.: Upper limb prosthesis use and abandonment: a survey of the last 25 years. Prosthet. Orthot. Int. **31**, 236–257 (2007). https://doi.org/10.1080/03093640600994581
15. Cordella, F., et al.: Literature review on needs of upper limb prosthesis users (2016). https://doi.org/10.3389/fnins.2016.00209
16. Biomedical Health and Research Program (BIOMED II) of the European Union: SENIAM. http://www.seniam.org/. Accessed 01 June 2018
17. Paiva, A., Ferreira, F., Catarino, A., Carvalho, M., Carvalho, H.: Design and characterization of a textile extension sensor for sports and health applications. In: IOP Conference Series: Materials Science and Engineering, vol. 459, p. 6 (2018). https://doi.org/10.1088/1757-899X/459/1/012058
18. Delagi, E.F., Iazzetti, J., Perotto, A.O., Morrison, D.: Anatomical Guide for the Electromyographer: The Limbs and Trunk. Charles C Thomas Publisher Ltd., New York (2011)
19. Kamen, G., Gabriel, D.A.: Essentials of Electromyography. Human Kinects, Leeds (2009)
20. Konrad, P.: The ABC of EMG. A Practical Introduction to Kinesiological Electromyography, pp. 1–60. Noraxon Inc., Scottsdale (2005). https://doi.org/10.1016/j.jacc.2008.05.066
21. Amrutha, N., Arul, V.H.: A review on noises in EMG signal and its removal. Int. J. Sci. Res. Publ. **7**, 23 (2017)
22. Chowdhury, R.H., Reaz, M.B.I., Bin Mohd Ali, M.A., Bakar, A.A.A., Chellappan, K., Chang, T.G.: Surface electromyography signal processing and classification techniques. Sens. (Switz.) **13**, 12431–12466 (2013). https://doi.org/10.3390/s130912431
23. Winter, D.A.: Biomechanics and Motor Control of Human Movement. Wiley, New York (2009)

Design of a Smart Mechatronic System to Combine Garments for Blind People: First Insights

Daniel Rocha[1(✉)], Vítor Carvalho[1,2], Filomena Soares[1], and Eva Oliveira[2]

[1] Algoritmi R&D, University of Minho, Guimarães, Portugal
id8057@alunos.uminho.pt, fsoares@dei.uminho.pt
[2] 2Ai, School of Technology, IPCA, Barcelos, Portugal
{vcarvalho,eoliveira}@ipca.pt

Abstract. In some professions, the way we dress, has a great impact in the context we are inserted. This task can be a huge problem specially for the visually impaired. They dependent on their relatives, friends, and/or support center professionals for the purchase or for choosing the clothes to wear. With the advance of technology, it is important to minimize the limitations of a blind person. One of the issues that remain to be explored is the case of the selection and combination of garments by a blind user. This paper aims to present a prototype to help blind people in the selection of garments.

Keywords: Smart closet · Mechatronic system · Machine learning · Combination clothes · Blind people

1 Introduction

In day-to-day life, visual impaired people find several difficulties that they try to manage and overcome the best way they can. Presently, society is being endowed with social, psychological and technological capacity to assist citizens with disabilities. Technology has brought new insights in solving, at least, some of these difficulties. Nevertheless, there are still some gaps to fulfill. Aesthetics is one example. In some professions, the way we dress, for example, has a great impact in the context we are inserted. This task can be a huge problem especially for the visually impaired. They dependent on their relatives, friends, and/or support center professionals for the purchase or for choosing the clothes to wear.

This project follows a previous work, "MyEyes" [1–3]. With the support of the Association of the Blind and Amblyopes of Portugal (ACAPO) [4] and the Association of Support for the Visually Impaired of Braga (AADVDB) [5].

The goal of this project is to assist the visually impaired in selecting the color combination of the clothes to wear through the development of a mechatronic system endowed with artificial intelligence to support the choice.

This paper in divided in 5 sections. Section 2 describe the previous and related work, in Sect. 3 mentions system goals, in Sect. 4 is described the prototype development and finally in Sect. 5 concludes with final remarks.

Technological developments have reached important proportions in terms of support for visually impaired. In this way, this paper presents some solutions to identify the highlights and the gaps that can be overcome.

There are various versions of smart virtual closets that have been applied in the current market. However, despite the different versions of virtual wardrobes there was no study on the consumers' attitudes [6].

In order to overcome this gap, Perry [6] performed and published a study on the intention of adoption of consumers of smart virtual cabinets. In this study a positive attitude towards smart virtual cabinets was led by two beliefs about the product, utility and ease of use. Utility and ease of use accounted for 84% of the variation in consumer attitudes towards the smart virtual closet. The results confirmed that the high utility of the product is one of the decisive factors of people's attitude towards intelligent virtual cabinets, and the low complexity of the operating system is a significant secondary determinant of consumer attitudes.

Recently, Bhowmick and Hazarik [7] published a survey, where 3010 papers were collected focused on the vision of assisted technology for visually impaired and future research trends. In conclusion, the authors emphasize the importance of the technological advance dedicated to blind people, referring to the increase in the functionality of the mobile technologies, advances in computational vision processing algorithms, miniaturization of electronic devices and the new cutting-edge medical interventions that should boost this field for the challenges and reality of successful technology creation.

Some fashion apps have been developed as STYLEBOOK, an application to manage the clothes, create outfits, and plan what to wear during the month [8]. Mode-Relier application [9] is another example that takes into account the skin-tone, hair color and even make up products. ShopStyle [10], allows to plan purchases based on the user favorite's stores, searching items across the web. Tailor [11] is a closet that learns the user's preferences and choices and suggests the combinations to wear. This system uses sensors called 'TailorTags' which are embedded in the clothes in order to detect the items and keep tracking of daily choses, learning and make suggestions [11].

A recommendation system based on semantic content to advise clothing items for recycling was proposed in [12]. In order to demonstrate the validity of its approach, an evaluation was performed on a set of data taken from the Web.

Goh et al. [13] present a smart wardrobe system, based on Radio Frequency Identification (RFID) technology where tags are placed on clothes in order to be identified by the mobile device.

Finally, another study proposes a system for the recognition of patterns in clothes and the dominant color in each image. The system is finger-based camera that allows users to query clothing colors and patterns by touch [14].

With regard to electronic devices, the Colorino, has come to fill the difficulties of the blind in the distinction of colors for the most varied tasks, since it helps in the choice of clothes, the washing procedure and the color combination [15].

There is also the ColorTest 2000, which is a device similar to Colorino that, like this one, does the identification of the colors, but also can read the dates and hours and detects if a light of the house is on or off [16].

Although there has been a great effort to develop systems to aid visual impaired, there is yet no solution capable of covering all the questions proposed in the scope of this project, namely an automatic system for combining and identifying the state of pieces of clothing for the visually impaired.

Thus, the scope of research presented in this paper has two modules: the first one is focused in algorithm of image processing and machine learning that will complement this second, presented in this paper, the mechatronic system. The algorithm will be the base of all system and has been developed in sense to be flexible for be adapted to other future situations. There are some projects that has been taking in account to develop our model [17–36].

In this context, the goal is to develop a physical prototype able to identify garments, colors, patterns having the ability to make autonomous fabric suggestions of clothing combinations for the user.

2   Related Work

There are various versions of smart virtual closets that have been applied in the current market. However, despite the different versions of virtual wardrobes there was no study on the consumers' attitudes [6].

In order to overcome this gap, Perry [6] performed and published a study on the intention of adoption of consumers of smart virtual cabinets. In this study a positive attitude towards smart virtual cabinets was led by two beliefs about the product, utility and ease of use. Utility and ease of use accounted for 84% of the variation in consumer attitudes towards the smart virtual closet. The results confirmed that the high utility of the product is one of the decisive factors of people's attitude towards intelligent virtual cabinets, and the low complexity of the operating system is a significant secondary determinant of consumer attitudes.

Recently, Bhowmick and Hazarik [7] published a survey, where 3010 papers were collected focused on the vision of assisted technology for visually impaired and future research trends. In conclusion, the authors emphasize the importance of the techno-logical advance dedicated to blind people, referring to the increase in the functionality of the mobile technologies, advances in computational vision processing algorithms, miniaturization of electronic devices and the new cutting-edge medical interventions that should boost this field for the challenges and reality of successful technology creation.

Some fashion apps have been developed as STYLEBOOK, an application to manage the clothes, create outfits, and plan what to wear during the month [8]. Mode-Relier application [9] is another example that takes into account the skin-tone, hair color and even make up products. ShopStyle [10], allows to plan purchases based on the user favorite's stores, searching items across the web. Tailor [11] is a closet that learns the user's preferences and choices and suggests the combinations to wear. This system uses sensors called 'TailorTags' which are embedded in the clothes in order to detect the items and keep tracking of daily choses, learning and make suggestions [11].

A recommendation system based on semantic content to advise clothing items for recycling was proposed in [12]. In order to demonstrate the validity of its approach, an evaluation was performed on a set of data taken from the Web.

Goh et al. [13] present a smart wardrobe system, based on Radio Frequency Identification (RFID) technology where tags are placed on clothes in order to be identified by the mobile device.

Finally, another study proposes a system for the recognition of patterns in clothes and the dominant color in each image. The system is finger-based camera that allows users to query clothing colors and patterns by touch [14].

With regard to electronic devices, the Colorino, has come to fill the difficulties of the blind in the distinction of colors for the most varied tasks, since it helps in the choice of clothes, the washing procedure and the color combination [15].

There is also the ColorTest 2000, which is a device similar to Colorino that, like this one, does the identification of the colors, but also can read the dates and hours and detects if a light of the house is on or off [16].

Although there has been a great effort to develop systems to aid visual impaired, there is yet no solution capable of covering all the questions proposed in the scope of this project, namely an automatic system for combining and identifying the state of pieces of clothing for the visually impaired.

Thus, the scope of research presented in this paper has two modules: the first one is focused in algorithm of image processing and machine learning that will complement this second, presented in this paper, the mechatronic system. The algorithm will be the base of all system and has been developed in sense to be flexible for be adapted to other future situations. There are some projects that has been taking in account to develop our model [17–36].

In this context, the goal is to develop a physical prototype able to identify garments, colors, patterns having the ability to make autonomous fabric suggestions of clothing combinations for the user.

3   System Goals

This work has as main objective which is the development of a low cost system, capable of supporting the visually impaired in performing the tests of inspection, identification and combination of garments.

In order to achieve this goal, specific objectives were set, in particular:

- Development of an algorithm for image acquisition, processing and analysis;
- Based on the previous algorithm, it is intended to develop software that is intuitive, easy to use, respecting accessibility rules;
- Development of artificial intelligence algorithms for combinations, suggestions and learning of the user's preferences;
- Building a database for storing all the information that will support artificial intelligence algorithms;

- Development of a mechatronic system for garment inspection;
- Construction of a physical prototype to prove the methodology and project developed.

In pursuit of the objectives, the following research question arises:

- How can a mechatronic device with artificial intelligence make the inspection, identification, combination and management of clothing for a blind person?

4 Prototype Development

The development of this prototype should consider parameters, as dimensions, response time, illumination and interface, among others.

4.1 Assumptions

For the scope of this work, it is assumed that clothing manufacturers embedded Near Field Communication (NFC) tags in their garments, at the time they are produced, where their characteristics such as: type, color, size, season, washing process and pattern are saved.

The prototype uses a Near Field Communication (NFC) reader to recognize it automatically (see Fig. 1).

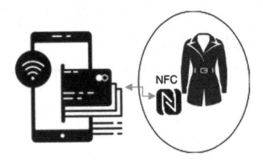

Fig. 1. NFC tag embedded in clothing able to be read.

The system was designed in sense that any device could be in touch with the smart closet. In this sense, the smart closet and all the devices are connected via the Internet.

4.2 Illumination

In an artificial vision application, its viability depends on the lighting factor.

The dark field is an annular illumination system perpendicular to the camera's capture axis. This technique is used to highlight surface defects or codes recorded on a surface.

The backlight are panels of homogeneous and diffuse light usually rectangular in shape. They are usually used by placing the part to be examined between the illumination and the camera, allowing to recognize the silhouette of an opaque object by contrast. There are many applications that require diffused lighting, which eliminates any kind of reflection; depending on the applications it can be used: coaxial lighting system, dome or diffuse low-relief lighting systems.

In order to achieve a homogeneous light field a light diffusion plate is used (see Fig. 2). A diffused illumination is used to reflect the properties of the clothing on the camera.

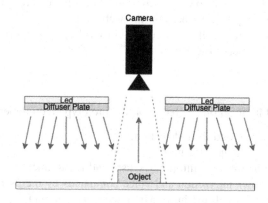

Fig. 2. Diffused illumination.

4.3   Smart Closet Features

In order to minimize hardware costs, the image processing and artificial intelligence algorithm will be processed in a centralized unit, cloud server.

Focused only on a smart closet, there are features that will be available and present in prototype projection like:

- Identify the garment and check the condition, whether it is wrinkled, dirty or ready for use;
- Save user feedback of clothing, meaning the rating of clothe combination;
- Compare its initial state with actual moment in order to recognize some degradation;
- dentify color for possible mistakes occurred during wash that have leads its changed.

4.4   Human - Machine Interface (HMI) Accessibility

This system will interact with the user and the Web application is the most usable way, since it could be access in anywhere. However, as the users are blind we need to provide mechanisms to assure proper accessibility requirements as users need to access the data by smartphone, or other device, even a tactile screen which is only possible through a combination of software and hardware.

The accessibility is an important factor with regard to the use of devices by people with visual impairments.

A study was performed [37] to help systematize research on visual impairments and mobile touchscreen interaction by providing an overview of the major causes of visual impairments that affect the effectiveness of touchscreen interaction and efficiency in smart mobile devices.

Other research refers to the opposing differences regarding the usability and aesthetics of Web content. Web aesthetics are found to increase purchase intent and search activation. Although web usability has a stronger effect on the purchase intention than the aesthetics of the web [38].

The W3C (World Wide Web Consortium) mentions the requirements to be fulfilled in the realization of graphic interfaces on the web [39].

In this way, our system will assure all usability rules, in interaction with a user in order to provide a total user-friendly system.

4.5   Hardware

The hardware, and its functions, is based on the prototype requirements and includes:

- Camera - color, state and dirty detection;
- Speaker - report all output for user by sound;
- Display - could be used for informative user and replacement of smartphone;
- Microphone - allows interaction and voice commands by the user;
- NFC Reader - readout all the information about the garment;
- DC Motor - allows to rotate the garment inside the closet;
- Braille Buttons - essential for inputs, like confirmation, feedback and start interaction by user.

In this way, the prototype besides being possible to pair with the smartphone will contain features that can be used separately. Thus, the prototype is accessible to all users, even those who do not want to use smartphones as an interface.

The unit controller chosen was Raspberry Pi (see Fig. 3). It is a small computer integrated in a single plate. Its versatility and low price allow it to be used in countless ways.

Its characteristics include [40]:

- Broadcom BCM2837B0, Cortex-A53 (ARMv8) 64-bit SoC @ 1.4 GHz;
- 1 GB LPDDR2 SDRAM;
- 2.4 GHz and 5 GHz IEEE 802.11.b/g/n/ac wireless LAN, Bluetooth 4.2, BLE;
- Gigabit Ethernet over USB 2.0 (maximum throughput 300 Mbps);
- Extended 40-pin GPIO header;
- Full-size HDMI;
- 4 USB 2.0 ports;
- CSI camera port for connecting a Raspberry Pi camera;
- DSI display port for connecting a Raspberry Pi touchscreen display;
- 4-pole stereo output and composite video port;
- Micro SD port for loading your operating system and storing data;

- 5 V/2.5 A DC power input;
- Power-over-Ethernet (PoE) support (requires separate PoE HAT).

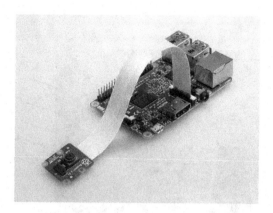

Fig. 3. Raspberry Pi and camera module [40].

In addition, it is possible to incorporate one of its two cameras, which provide sufficient features for a first exploration of image acquisition. The characteristics of camera v2 can be found in Table 1.

Table 1. Camera module v2.

Still resolution	8 Megapixels
Weight	3 g
Sensor	Sony IMX219
Sensor resolution	3280 × 2464 pixels
Sensor image area	3.68 × 2.76 mm (4.6 mm diagonal)
Pixel size	1.12 μm × 1.12 μm
Optical size	1/4″

4.6   Prototype Dimensions

The prototype should have, at least, the following dimensions:

- Height: 180 cm;
- Width: 130 cm;

These dimensions took into account the Horizontal Field of View (HFOV) of the camera as well the vertical. By this way Eq. (1) show the trigonometry equation to calculate the dimensions based in FOV of camera.

$$HFOV[mm] = 2 \times OD[mm] \times \tan(AFOV[degrees]/2) \qquad (1)$$

Where the distance to object (OD) from the camera as well the Angle of Field of View is necessary to obtain the horizontal distance, as well as, vertical distance.

The first version of the proposed prototype is presented below (see Fig. 4).

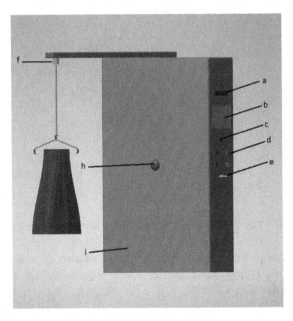

Fig. 4. Proposal prototype – smart closet. a - Speaker; b - Display; c - Microphone; d - Braille Buttons; e - NFC Reader; f - DC Motor; h - Camera; i - Led panel for illumination.

In summary, the prototype of the smart closet has a back panel with led diffusing light that allows homogeneous light, where in the middle of the panel is placed a camera that will take photos in order to inspect the garment.

In the side of light panel, the user is able to interact with the smart closet by voice and receive output by the speaker. The NFC reader can collect all information from clothing tag and associate to the database its characteristics.

In order to inspect the two sides of the garment a motor is placed in order to rotate it.

The buttons in braille allows the user to interact with the system. The smartphone can also be connected with the closet allowing to control the system.

The system is connected to a cloud server that is responsible for processing the information. The system is connected to a cloud server that is responsible for processing the information relative to image processing and machine learning. By this way, the data processing is centralized and consequently the costs associated to the hardware integration with high capacity to handling the data are avoided.

This design takes into account the fact that we want to control the clothes in a controlled environment.

5   Final Remarks

It is important to recognize that clothing aesthetics are of central importance in the life of blind people, who are happily increasingly inserted in the labor market, have an active social life, and as with most people in the same circumstances, they need to be accepted and recognized.

A duly qualified or rehabilitated blind person has all the conditions to, if he/she wishes, be able to live alone or even to have a marital relationship with another blind person. However, blind people experience some difficulties with regard to clothing. Some are overcome with the help of family or friends, others with a great organizational capacity.

In order to select and match the clothes the person wears daily, it is crucial to have a faultless organization and internal discipline. During the purchase of the garment, the blind person asks the other person for help in describing the garment with as much information as possible, in order to distinguish from the other garments, basically looking for something different, such as a tag, a different area, a cutout, deep down the idea is to find a distinct brand in the clothe.

The next step is to organize the different types and colors of clothes in drawers and drawers, in order to become easier to pick up a particular piece that it is intended to wear that day. However, such a thorough process can be prone to errors, particularly when washing clothes and having to replace them where they are removed, or when using luggage, where the organization is extraordinarily more difficult.

Another difficulty is to detect dirt or stains on clothing. Except for situations where stains can be detected by touch, for the most parts this is objectively impossible.

Against this backdrop of some difficulties, technology can be a very interesting ally in which a smart wardrobe would be welcomed.

Thus, the mechatronic system proposed aims to help blind people to overcome their difficulty in choosing clothes. So, this system proposes a new concept for significantly improve the daily of the blind, allowing the blind to combine garments, identifying dirt and garments that are not in good condition. Moreover, the user could benefit from the automatic suggestions resulting from the machine learning algorithms.

This first prototype also intends to evaluate the interaction of the user with the system and verify the effects in terms of well-being and self-esteem, resulting from greater autonomy of the blind.

Acknowledgment. This work has the support of Association of the Blind and Amblyopes of Portugal (ACAPO) and Association of Support for the Visually Impaired of Braga (AADVDB). Their considerations gave (and still give) this project the first insights to a viable solution for the blind people community. This work has been supported by national funds through FCT – Fundação para a Ciência e Tecnologia within the Project Scope: UID/CEC/00319/2019.

References

1. Rocha, D., Carvalho, V., Oliveira, E., Goncalves, J., Azevedo, F.: MyEyes - automatic combination system of clothing parts to blind people: first insights. In: 2017 IEEE 5th International Conference on Serious Games and Applications for Health (SeGAH), pp. 1–5 (2017)
2. Rocha, D., Carvalho, V., Oliveira, E.: MyEyes - automatic combination system of clothing parts to blind people: prototype validation. In: SENSORDEVICES 2017 Conference, Rome, Italy, 10–14 September 2017 (2017)
3. Rocha, D., Carvalho, V., Gonçalves, J., Azevedo, F., Oliveira, E.: Development of an automatic combination system of clothing parts for blind people: MyEyes. Sens. Transducers **219**(1), 26–33 (2018)
4. ACAPO - Associação dos Cegos e Amblíopes de Portugal. http://www.acapo.pt/. Accessed 22 June 2019
5. AADVDB - Associação de Apoio aos Deficientes Visuais do Distrito de Braga. https://aadvdb.pt/. Accessed 22 June 2019
6. Perry, A.: Consumers' acceptance of smart virtual closets. J. Retail. Consum. Serv. **33**, 171–177 (2016)
7. Bhowmick, A., Hazarika, S.M.: An insight into assistive technology for the visually impaired and blind people: state-of-the-art and future trends. J. Multimodal User Interfaces **11**(2), 149–172 (2017)
8. Stylebook Closet App: A closet and wardrobe fashion app for the iPhone, iPad and iPod. http://www.stylebookapp.com/index.html. Accessed 21 June 2019
9. Mode-Relier: Secrets to look stylish everyday. https://www.mode-relier.com/. Accessed 21 June 2019
10. ShopStyle: Search and find the latest in fashion. https://www.shopstyle.com/. Accessed 21 June 2019
11. Tailor: The smart closet. http://www.tailortags.com/. Accessed 21 June 2019
12. Kolstad, A., Ozgobek, O., Gulla, J.A., Litlehamar, S.: Content-based recommendations for sustainable wardrobes using linked open data. Mob. Netw. Appl. **23**(6), 1727–1734 (2018)
13. Goh, K.N., Chen, Y.Y., Lin, E.S.: Developing a smart wardrobe system. In: 2011 IEEE Consumer Communications and Networking Conference (CCNC), pp. 303–307 (2011)
14. Stearns, L., Findlater, L., Froehlich, J.E.: Applying transfer learning to recognize clothing patterns using a finger-mounted camera. In: 20th International ACM SIGACCESS Conference on Computers and Accessibility, pp. 349–351 (2018)
15. Colorino Color Identifier - Light Detector - Assistive Technology at Easter Seals Crossroads. https://www.eastersealstech.com/2016/07/05/colorinos-color-identifier-light-detector/. Accessed 19 Feb 2019
16. Colortest Standard - Computer Room Services. https://www.comproom.co.uk/product/colortest-classic/. Accessed 19 Feb 2019
17. Jafari-Khouzani, K., Soltanian-Zadeh, H.: Radon transform orientation estimation for rotation invariant texture analysis. IEEE Trans. Pattern Anal. Mach. Intell. **27**(6), 1004–1008 (2005)
18. Cheng, C.-I., Liu, D.S.-M.: An intelligent clothes search system based on fashion styles. In: 2008 International Conference on Machine Learning and Cybernetics, vol. 3, p. 1592 (2008)
19. Kita, Y., Ueshiba, T., Neo, E.S., Kita, N.: Clothes state recognition using 3D observed data. In: 2009 IEEE International Conference on Robotics and Automation, ICRA 2009, p. 1220 (2009)
20. Yuan, S., Tian, Y.: Rotation and illumination invariant texture analysis: matching clothes with complex patterns for blind people. In: 2010 3rd International Congress on Image and Signal Processing, pp. 2643–2647 (2010)

21. Yang, M., Yu, K.: Real-time clothing recognition in surveillance videos. In: 2011 18th IEEE International Conference on Image Processing (ICIP), pp. 2937–2940 (2011)
22. Yuan, S., Tian, Y., Arditi, A.: Clothing matching for visually impaired persons. Technol. Disabil. 23(2), 75–85 (2011)
23. Zheng, X., Liu, N.: Color recognition of clothes based on k-means and mean shift. In: 2012 IEEE International Conference on Intelligent Control, Automatic Detection and High-End Equipment (ICADE), pp. 49–53 (2012)
24. Yamaguchi, K., Kiapour, M.H., Ortiz, L.E., Berg, T.L.: Parsing clothing in fashion photographs. In: 2012 IEEE Conference on Computer Vision and Pattern Recognition (CVPR), pp. 3570–3577 (2012)
25. Liu, S., et al.: Fashion parsing with weak color-category labels. IEEE Trans. Multimed. 16 (1), 253–265 (2014)
26. Manfredi, M., Grana, C., Calderara, S., Cucchiara, R.: A complete system for garment segmentation and color classification. Mach. Vis. Appl. 25(4), 955–969 (2014)
27. Cheng, C.-I., Liu, D.S.-M., Liu, M.-L., Wan, I.-E.: Clothing matchmaker: automatically finding apposite garment pairs from personal wardrobe. Int. J. Organ. Innov. 7(1), 79–104 (2014)
28. Yang, X., Yuan, S., Tian, Y.: Assistive clothing pattern recognition for visually impaired people. IEEE Trans. Hum. Mach. Syst. 44(2), 234–243 (2014)
29. Jarin Joe Rini, J., Thilagavathi, B.: Recognizing clothes patterns and colours for blind people using neural network. In: 2015 IEEE International Conference on Innovations in Information, Embedded and Communication Systems, ICIIECS 2015 (2015)
30. Surakarin, W., Chongstitvatana, P.: Predicting types of clothing using SURF and LDP based on bag of features. In: 2015 12th International Conference on Electrical Engineering/ Electronics, Computer, Telecommunications and Information Technology, ECTI-CON 2015 (2015)
31. Yamaguchi, K., Kiapour, M.H., Ortiz, L.E., Berg, T.L.: Retrieving similar styles to parse clothing. IEEE Trans. Pattern Anal. Mach. Intell. 37(5), 1028–1040 (2015)
32. Jarin Joe Rini, J., Thilagavathi, B.: Recognizing clothes patterns and colours for blind people using neural network. In: 2015 International Conference on Innovations in Information, Embedded and Communication Systems (ICIIECS), pp. 1–5 (2015)
33. Liu, Z., Luo, P., Qiu, S., Wang, X., Tang, X.: DeepFashion: powering robust clothes recognition and retrieval with rich annotations. In: 2016 IEEE Conference on Computer Vision and Pattern Recognition (CVPR), pp. 1096–1104 (2016)
34. Liang, X., Lin, L., Yang, W., Luo, P., Huang, J., Yan, S.: Clothes co-parsing via joint image segmentation and labeling with application to clothing retrieval. IEEE Trans. Multimed. 18 (6), 1175 (2016)
35. Wazarkar, S., Keshavamurthy, B.N.: Fashion image classification using matching points with linear convolution. Multimed. Tools Appl. 77(19), 25941–25958 (2018)
36. Kashilani, D., Damahe, L.B., Thakur, N.V.: An overview of image recognition and retrieval of clothing items. In: 2018 International Conference on Research in Intelligent and Computing in Engineering (RICE), pp. 1–6 (2018)
37. Vatavu, R.-D.: Visual impairments and mobile touchscreen interaction: state-of-the-art, causes of visual impairment, and design guidelines. Int. J. Hum. Comput. Interact. 33(6), 486–509 (2017)
38. Wang, Y.J., Lou, H., Hong, S.: Beautiful beyond useful? The role of web aesthetics. J. Comput. Inf. Syst. 50(3), 121–129 (2010)
39. Accessibility - W3C. https://www.w3.org/standards/webdesign/accessibility.html. Accessed 28 June 2019
40. Buy a Raspberry Pi 3 Model B+ – Raspberry Pi. https://www.raspberrypi.org/products/raspberry-pi-3-model-b-plus/. Accessed 22 June 2019

IoT for Health Applications
and Solutions

Towards a Smartwatch for Cuff-Less Blood Pressure Measurement Using PPG Signal and Physiological Features

Franck Mouney[1,2]([✉]), Teodor Tiplica[1], Magid Hallab[2], Mickeal Dinomais[1], and Jean-Baptiste Fasquel[1]

[1] LARIS Laboratory, Angers University, Angers, France
mouney.franck@gmail.com
[2] Axelife SAS, Saint-Nicolas-de-Redon, France

Abstract. The context of this work concerns the development of a connected smartwatch for the continuous daily monitoring of physiological parameters to prevent cardiovascular diseases, and for the follow-up of the efficiency of treatments, against hypertension for example. This paper focuses on a particular parameter, the blood pressure (BP), to be automatically measured from the Photoplethysmogram (PPG) signal, to be acquired using a smartwatch. The proposed method is based on the automatic pulse wave detection from the PPG signal. Then, using the Lasso algorithm, a relation has been established between the blood pressure and the spectral representation of the normalized pulse wave, combined with other physiological information (age, body mass index and hear rate). The proposed method has been evaluated on a recent large public database of 219 subjects, covering a large range of ages (20–89), body mass indices and of blood pressures. Experimental results show acceptable performances in terms of accuracy. Compared to a recent related work depicting a slightly lower estimation error, a strength of our approach regards its robustness with respect to the signal quality, this being crucial for a use in daily routine in real IoT conditions, as it is the case in this context of smartwatch.

Keywords: Photoplethysmogram (PPG) · Blood pressure (BP) · FFT · Lasso · IoT

1 Introduction

During the last 15 years, a lot of research has been made on photoplethysmography signal (PPG). In 1996, [1] evaluated morphological changes of the pulse wave due to ventilation, anaesthesia, etc... Moreover, this study also underlined the relevance of analyzing peripheral pulse wave in cardiac function, for diagnosis purpose. Since then, some research has been focused on predicting arterial blood pressure thanks to PPG signal as it would allow non-invasive

N. M. Garcia et al. (Eds.): HealthyIoT 2019, LNICST 314, pp. 67–76, 2020.
https://doi.org/10.1007/978-3-030-42029-1_5

and continuous monitoring. Coupling PPG monitoring with Internet of Things (IoT) application could provide to the doctor real-time measurement and trends over weeks of patient's blood pressure. This would allow the early detection of hypertension, as well as the follow-up of the efficiency of the anti-hypertension treatment, therefore facilitating its adaptation [2,3]. In many ways, this kind of technology would help to improve healthcare system.

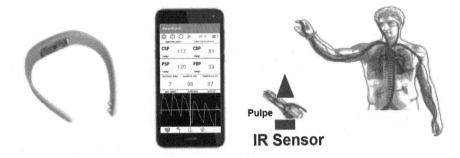

Fig. 1. Smartwatch, IoT and pulse wave. Left: Developed smartwatch and mobile application. Right: Infrared (IR) sensor on the wirst to acquire PPG signal.

This work takes place within the context of the development of a smartwatch iHeartWatch with Axelife which is able to record several physiological parameters, including PPG signal, from wirst. This smartwatch is connected to a smartphone itself connected to the web. The longterm goal is to provide predictive data analysis to improve patient's cardiovascular diagnosis and thus help in decision making. In this context, the first challenge for the early detection of cardiovascular diseases is to monitor blood pressure over time thanks to PPG sensor, as illustrated by Fig. 1.

In this paper, the proposed approach is based on spectral signal analysis rather than on temporal features, that are assumed to be more tedious to acquire, and more sensitive to signal quality, as illustrated by recent works [4], ignoring some abnormal PPG signals. Similarly to [4], our approach exploits physiological features, this being often ignored by most other related methods. Note that this work has to be integrated in a more complex acquisition and signal processing system which should be able to contextualize and select admissible pulse waves.

Rest of the paper is organized as follows. Section 2 focuses on the description of the method used with the different processing steps. Section 3 describes the data and experimental results. Sections 4 and 5 respectively contains a discussion and a conclusion.

2   Method

The block-diagram in Fig. 2 provide an overview of the proposed approach, including several steps of signal processing that are described herebelow.

2.1 Pre-processing

Preprocessing is require to further exploit PPG signal. This first preliminary step is crucial, as underlined by related works dedicated to the study of filtering techniques on public databases [5,6]. In our work, preprocessing consists in several steps.

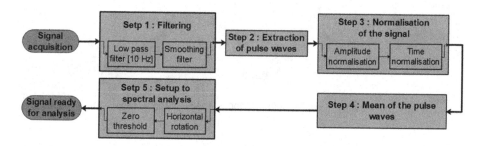

Fig. 2. Block-diagram of signal processing steps.

Step 1 - Filtering
We use a low pass linear-phase FIR filter to suppress high frequencies in the signal (Fig. 3B) with cuff-off frequency of 10 Hz which allows to suppress any power-line interference (50 Hz, 60 Hz, etc.). A smoothing is then applied by means of a digital filter with a polynomial order of three.

Step 2 - Extraction of pulse wave
Pulse wave extraction is achieved by searching for the minimal values between systolic peaks (Fig. 3C).

Step 3 - Normalisation of the signal in amplitude and time
Each extracted pulse wave has been normalized between 0 and 1, to focus on the shape of the wave, regardless to its amplitude. Then, time normalisation has been applied (length of pulse wave set to 1), to remove the dependency to the heart rate (and in particular to its variations over the set of pulse waves). Note that the heart rate is measured using another sensor (averaged measure over several cardiac cycle) (Fig. 4D).

Step 4 - Mean of pulse wave for each subject
Each signal embeds several pulse waves. To get a more robust blood pressure estimation, an averaged normalized pulse waves have been considered over all subject's signals (average over the set of detected pulse waves). Leading to a single mean pulse wave per subject (Fig. 4E).

Step 5 - Rotation and zero threshold
Last pre-processing step consisted in rotating the pulse wave horizontally and thus being able to perform zero padding in order to increase the spectral resolution (Fig. 4F).

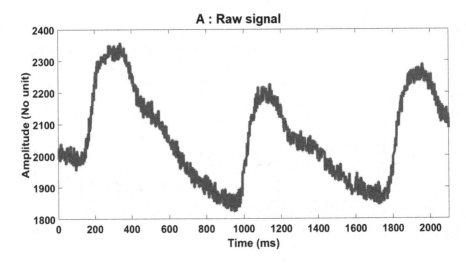

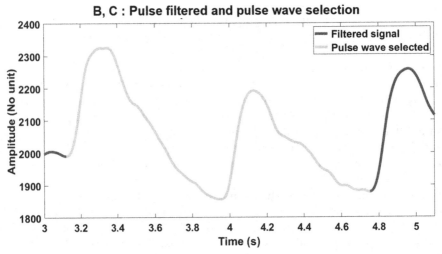

Fig. 3. Pre-processing steps of the PPG signal. A: Raw signal, B: Filtered signal, C: Selected pulse wave

2.2 Feature Extraction

Feature extraction is performed in the frequency domain (FFT). This choice enables to avoid the detection of specific keypoints in the time domain, as considered in [4], on which are extracted time-domain-based features. Note that we only consider spectrum coefficients ranging from 0 to 10 Hz (Fig. 5).

2.3 Lasso Algorithm

Lasso is a regression analysis method [7]. It is used in large problems resolution, when there is an important set of features potentially linked to a target

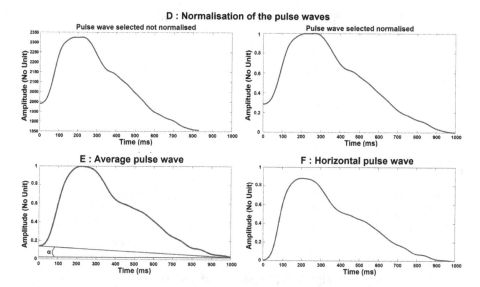

Fig. 4. Pre-processing steps of the PPG signal. D: Normalisation of pulse waves, E: Average pulse wave with alpha (α) the rotational angle to horizontal position, F: Horizontal pulse wave

value. This algorithm can perform a restricted selection of variables significantly connected the target value to make an accurate prediction. Lasso algorithm has been applied on following variables, including physiological ones (age, body mass index (BMI), heart rate) and those related to the PPG signal (spectral coefficients).

3 Experiments

For experiments, a public database [6] has been considered, with the underlying advantage of facilitating the comparison with third party works.

Data were collected at the People's Hospital of Guilin (PHG) in China [6] during a clinical laboratory measurement. It is composed of 657 PPG signals of 2.1 s each from 219 subjects (3 signals per subject). We end-up with a total of 212 pulse waves (one by subject) after the pre-processing steps. The 7 subjects missing is due to bad signal quality (mostly outliers for PHG database, see example Fig. 6B) that failed the automatic extraction of the pulse waves. It covers a large range of ages [20–89] and a large range of blood pressure too as its incorporates 3 types of hypertensive states. Furthermore, the database includes physiological information like height, weight, heart rate but also it contains an illness record about diabetes, cerebral infraction and cerebrovascular disease.

To establish a relationship between PPG waveforms and BP, the data acquisition procedure has been conducted in accordance with standard experimental

Figure A : Superposed pulse waves

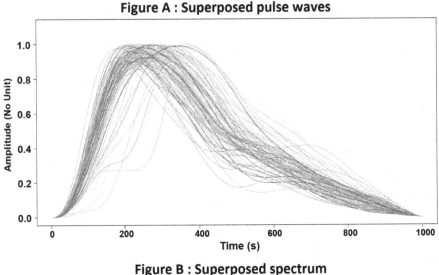

Figure B : Superposed spectrum

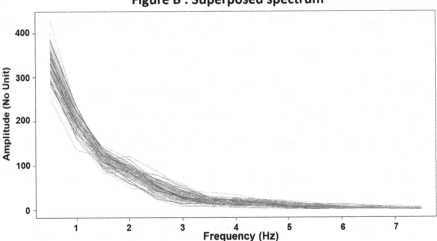

Fig. 5. A: Superposed pulse waves selected from database (colors, from blue to red, encode the hypertensive state, red corresponding to high hypertension). B: Superposed related spectrum magnitude of pulse wave with same color scale (Color figure online)

conditions. It is important to mention that each subject was sitting in a comfortable position for 10 min to reach a rest state which allows reliable non-invasive cuff-less and continuous PPG signal measurement. However, this database comprise one drawback, the duration of the signals is very short, 2.1 s. Note that there is no possibility to evaluate dynamic changes.

During the experimentation, Lasso algorithm gave us some specific frequencies to use as features in order to predict BP. Table 1 shows the spectral frequen-

cies and physiological characteristics selected to predict Systolic Blood Pressure
(SBP) and Diastolic Blood Pressure (DBP).

Table 1. Lasso selected features.

	DBP	SBP
Frequency (Hz)	1 - 3.5 - 5 - 9	0.5 - 1 - 2.5 - 4 - 8.5
Physiological characteristics	BMI - HR	Age - BMI - HR

Results of BP prediction performance are reported in Table 3. They are presented as Mean Absolute Error (MAE) and standard deviation (SD) of the MAE
in terms of millimeter of mercury (mmHg), this being the standard unit for blood
pressure in medicine. Formula are presented in Table 2. We computed K-fold
cross-validated mean squared prediction error to evaluate total efficiency of our
model.

Table 2. Evaluation performance formula.

$$\text{MAE} = \tfrac{1}{n} \sum_{t=1}^{n} |BP_{predicted} - BP_{reference}|$$

$$\text{SD MAE} = \sqrt{\tfrac{1}{n} \sum_{t=1}^{n} (BP_{predicted} - MAE)}$$

According to [9], the criteria to fulfil AAMI protocol is that the mean difference and standard deviation between the given value of the mercury standard
device and the one of the test devices must be in within $5\,\text{mmHg} \pm 8\,\text{mmHg}$.
From this point of view, even if we do not use exactly the same performance
values, [4] seems closer to be accepted than us as long as their is a control on
signal quality otherwise our algorithms will probably perform the same or better
on PHG database.

Table 3. Results: Blood pressure estimation error MAE (SD).

Method	DBP (mmHg)	SBP (mmHg)	Discarded subjects (%)
Yang2018	4.13 (5.26)	9.18 (12.57)	12.78
Our approach	7.98 (6.25)	13.69 (10.61)	3.20

We tried to compute pulse waves without normalisation in amplitude too but
results were a bit worse, therefore justifying our choice. In our sense, normalization is relevant due to environmental condition that can influence the signal

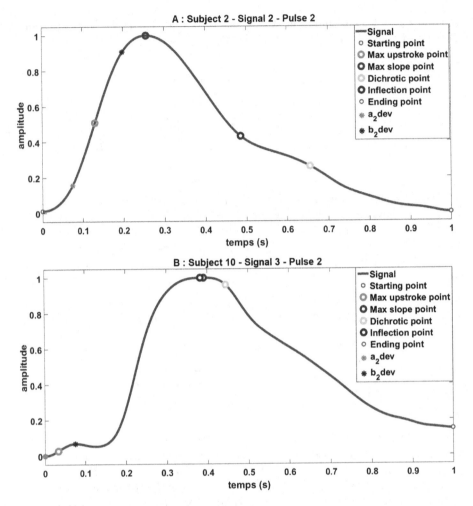

Fig. 6. Extraction of specific points on pulse wave. A: Correctly detected key points, B: Uncorrectly detected key points

amplitude measured. Especially due to temperature, lighting, skin contact quality, degree of pressure applied on the sensor against skin. All of those combined could influence estimation results if the pulse waves are not normalised.

Discarded subjects regards the proportion of the database that has been ignored. In our case, few subjects has been automatically discarded, while in [4], this has been done by visual control the signal quality. They do not give any explanation about the reason of ignoring these signals, nor any quantitative measure about the impact of the signals on the value of the MAE.

4   Discussion

The proposed method leads to acceptable performances in terms of MAE but appears more robust than [4]. Note that our results remain acceptable from a medical point of view, at least to provide an information about the evolution of the blood pressure in such a context of continuous daily monitoring using a smartwatch. The robustness regards to ability of our proposal to process all PPG signals, except the 7 cases which have been automatically discarded. In [4], about 13% of signals (i.e. 4 times more) have been ignored. Moreover, it must be underlined that these irrelevant signals have been manually discarded, based on a visual control of their quality. In our sense, it is crucial not to be too sensitive to signal quality or, at least, to be able to automatically detect irrelevant signals (this being done manually in [4]). This is particularly critical for a use in real conditions (smartwatch), which is not the case for the considered database where signals have been acquired in a controlled environment. This lack of robustness of [4] is probably due to the large number of temporal features to be extracted (12 features), each one with a dedicated algorithm focusing on the detection of some keypoints on the pulse wave. To illustrate this aspect, we have also implemented these features using the method described in [4]: Fig. 6 provides some examples of uncorrectly detected key points on some pulse waves. It has been observed that in many cases, keypoints were uncorrectly recovered, due to the variability of the signal. In our case, the observed robustness is probably due to the fact that, except for the step focusing on the pulse wave detection, our proposal is based on spectral representation of the signal (Fourier transform), and a straightforward measurement of the relation between this representation and the blood pressure (using the Lasso algorithm). Our work is only compared with [4] because of the considered database. Indeed, this recently published database is the only one providing, together with PPG signals, physiological information regarding subjects (this being not the case of other databases such as MIMIC [8]). Such an information has been proved to be required [4] to ensure a better estimation of the blood pressure.

5   Conclusion

IoT-based devices such as smartwatch are really promising systems for the non-invasive daily monitoring of the cardiovascular system in order to prevent diseases such as hypertension. A difficulty is the automatic and robust measurement of physiological parameters for a use in daily routine in real condition, with, for instance, lightening and temperature variations. The proposed method aims at providing such a robust estimation of the blood pressure from the PPG signal. Although providing a slightly larger error than a recent work on this topic, measurements remain useful to provide a trend of the evolution of the blood pressure in a non invasive manner. A strength of this method is its robustness with respect to the quality of the signal, and its ability to automatic ignore irrelevant waves, this being manually done in recent related works. Future steps will focus on the error reduction by integrating other signal features and additional external physiological information.

References

1. Murray, W.B., Foster, P.A.: The peripheral pulse wave: information overlooked. J. Clin. Monit. **12**(5), 365–377 (1996)
2. Perloff, D., Sokolow, M., Cowan, R.: The prognostic value of ambulatory blood pressures. JAMA **249**(20), 2792–2798 (1983)
3. Perloff, D., Sokolow, M., Cowan, R.: The prognostic value of ambulatory blood pressure monitoring in treated hypertensive patients. J. Hypertens. Suppl.: Official J. Int. Soc. Hypertens. **9**(1), S33-9 (1991)
4. Yang, S., Zhang, Y., Cho, S.Y., Morgan, S.P., Correia, R., Wen, L.: Cuff-less blood pressure measurement using fingertip photoplethysmogram signals and physiological characteristics. In: Optics in Health Care and Biomedical Optics VIII, vol. 10820, p. 1082036. International Society for Optics and Photonics, October 2018
5. Liang, Y., Elgendi, M., Chen, Z., Ward, R.: An optimal filter for short photoplethysmogram signals. Sci. Data **5**, 180076 (2018)
6. Liang, Y., Chen, Z., Liu, G., Elgendi, M.: A new, short-recorded photoplethysmogram dataset for blood pressure monitoring in China. Sci. Data **5**, 180020 (2018)
7. Efron, B., Hastie, T., Johnstone, I., Tibshirani, R.: Least angle regression. Ann. Stat. **32**(2), 407–499 (2004)
8. Goldberger, A.L., et al.: PhysioBank, PhysioToolkit, and PhysioNet: components of a new research resource for complex physiologic signals. Circulation **101**(23), e215–e220 (2000)
9. O'Brien, E., Waeber, B., Parati, G., Staessen, J., Myers, M.G.: Blood pressure measuring devices: recommendations of the European Society of Hypertension. BMJ **322**(7285), 531–536 (2001)

Wi-Fi-Enabled Automatic Eating Moment Monitoring Using Smartphones

Zhenzhe Lin[1(✉)], Yucheng Xie[2], Xiaonan Guo[2], Chen Wang[3], Yanzhi Ren[4], and Yingying Chen[1]

[1] WINLAB, Rutgers University, New Brunswick, NJ 08901, USA
zhenzhe.lin@rutgers.edu, yingche@scarletmail.rutgers.edu
[2] Indiana University-Purdue University Indianapolis, Indianapolis, IN 46202, USA
{yx11,xg6}@iupui.edu
[3] Louisiana State University, Baton Rouge, LA 70803, USA
chenwang1@lsu.edu
[4] University of Electronic Science and Technology of China, Chengdu 611731, People's Republic of China
renyanzhi05@uestc.edu.cn

Abstract. Dietary habits are closely correlated with people's health. Study reveals that unhealthy eating habits may cause various diseases such as obesity, diabetes and anemia. To help users create good eating habits, eating moment monitoring plays a significant role. However, traditional methods mainly rely on manual self-report or wearable devices, which either require much user efforts or intrusive dedicated hardware. In this work, we propose a user effort-free eating moment monitoring system by leveraging the WiFi signals extracted from the commercial off-the-shelf (COTS) smartphones. In particular, our system captures the eating activities of users to determine the eating moments. The proposed system can further identify the fine-grained food intake gestures (e.g., eating with fork, knife, spoon, chopsticks and bard hand) to estimate the detailed eating episode for each food intake gesture. Utilizing the dietary information, our system shows the potential to infer the food category and food amount. Extensive experiments with 10 subjects over 400-min eating show that our system can recognize a user's food intake gestures with up to 97.8% accuracy and estimate the dietary moment within 1.1-s error.

Keywords: Eating moment monitoring · WiFi sensing · Healthy eating

1 Introduction

Dietary behavior is an important factor of healthy eating and is closely related to the health condition of an individual. Due to the increasing stress at work and the fast-paced lifestyle in the modern society, people tend to form unhealthy

© ICST Institute for Computer Sciences, Social Informatics and Telecommunications Engineering 2020
Published by Springer Nature Switzerland AG 2020. All Rights Reserved
N. M. Garcia et al. (Eds.): HealthyIoT 2019, LNICST 314, pp. 77–91, 2020.
https://doi.org/10.1007/978-3-030-42029-1_6

eating habits unconsciously, such as overeating and eating disorder, leading to weight-gain or obesity. Studies show that overweight and obesity are the most prevalent health problems, which further cause various diseases such as diabetes, high blood pressure, cardiovascular diseases and breathing disorder [1,2]. Recent survey by the World Health Organizations reveals that more than 1.9 billion adults are overweight and 650 million are obese [3], and they are suffering or under the risk of the various eating-related health problems. Therefore, it is crucial to provide an appropriate assistance to each individual for improving their dietary behaviors. To achieve this goal, we need to help the user to keep close track of every moment of his/her eating activities.

Eating moment monitoring provides the comprehensive dietary information to help users understand their eating behaviors (e.g., overeating, undereating, skipping meals, irregular eating schedules and eating too fast). Based on that, users could realize the overall health condition in regard to his/her eating behavior and further boost their ability to create and sustain a healthy lifestyle. Traditional eating moment or eating episode monitoring mainly rely on the self-reports including food questionnaires and meal records [4]. For example, a mobile application called ate [5] allows users to track their dietary information regarding the food category by capturing the food photos from cameras. However, self-report approaches require proactive participation and self-consciousness which seems to be obtrusive for the users. Moreover, these instruments suffer from subjective bias and memory imprecision [6]. To provide automatic eating moment monitoring without requiring much user efforts, recent studies propose to leverage the wearable devices worn on the user's ear [7] or wrist [8] for dietary activity recognition. Unfortunately, there are some limitations since the dedicated wearable devices also incur high-cost issues and bring additional uncomfortable user experience to individuals. Different from the above studies, in this work, we propose to leverage the WiFi signals extracted from the user's smartphones to provide fine-grained dietary moment monitoring. While eating, user can simply place his/her personal smartphone on the dining table, which automatically recognizes the food intake gestures to monitor the user's eating moments.

Recent years have witnessed the initial success of WiFi-based human activity sensing [9–11]. But in order to utilize the WiFi signals to automatically recognize the user's dietary moments, a number of challenges need to be addressed: (1) to monitor the user's eating moments, we need to recognize the user's eating activities from the many other daily activities. But it is hard for a smartphone to store a large activity profile covering all the user's daily activities such as typing, reading, sitting and stretching; (2) besides recognizing the coarse eating moments, fine-grained eating moment monitoring also require differentiating the user's various food intake gestures (e.g., eating with a folk, chopsticks or bare hand), which reflects the user's detailed eating behavior and information of the food. But the various eating gestures are similar and hard to be distinguished from the WiFi signals, which all involve the hand movements from the table to mouth; (3) using the WiFi signals from the smartphone to provide human activity recognition is still an open area. This is because the WiFi signals obtained by the smartphone is relatively weak and noisy due to the integrated small size of internal antennas.

To address these challenges, we propose a WiFi-enabled automatic dietary moment recognition system for assisting the individuals to improve dietary behaviors by using their own smartphones. We extract the Channel State Information (CSI) from the WiFi signals to capture the user's fine-grained eating activities and estimate the detailed eating moments, which is non-invasive to the user and does not require additional hardware. Specifically, we utilize a Fuzzy C-Means clustering method to distinguish the dietary activities from the many other human daily activities and detect the dietary moments based on deriving the CSI spectrogram. Moreover, we extract the unique features to capture the eating gestures' behavioral characteristics and further classify them based on the utensils held by the user (i.e., fork, knife, spoon, chopsticks and bare hand). In addition, we derive the starting and ending point of the eating moment for each eating gesture and estimate the duration and speed for meals.

Our Contributions Are Summarized as Follows:

- We demonstrate that the channel state information extracted from the WiFi signals can be used to provide fine-grained eating moment monitoring for the users, which can further interpret the user's eating behavior, including overeating, undereating, eating disorder and eating too fast.
- We develop a device-free dietary recognition system based on the WiFi signals to automatically track the user's eating activity, which can be easily deployed on the user's smartphone without incurring additional costs or changing the existing WiFi infrastructures.
- We adopt the Fuzzy C-means clustering technique to differentiate the dietary activities from all human daily activities. We then utilize different machine learning classification approaches (i.e., Random Forest, Naive Bayes, K Nearest Neighbors, Discriminant Analysis Classifier) to identify the food intake gestures based on the utensils held by users. Moreover, we propose an intake gesture density derivation method to calculate the comprehensive dietary moments and develop the ingestion period estimation method to derive the dietary moment statistics.
- Extensive experiments with 10 people over 400-min eating show that our system can recognize a user's food intake gestures with up to 97.8% accuracy and estimate the dietary moments within 1.1 s error.

2   Related Work

The exploit of dietary monitoring methods provokes the feasibility to infer the health condition of subjects based on eating. Traditional eating monitoring methods are mainly based on self-report or meal recalls. These methods require users to manual write down the start/end time of their eating activities on food diaries or fill questionnaires by recalling their memory [12]. The smartphone Apps allows the user to more flexibly record their meal by typing texts and taking photos [5].

But these self-report methods rely too much on the user's active participation and impose a memory burden. Thus these methods are obtrusive to the users and hard to obtain the timely precise eating monitoring result. Moreover, these methods suffer from the subjective bias and memory recall imprecision.

To reduce the user's efforts, the vision-based methods are developed to recognize eating activities automatically by utilizing the cameras to take photos or videos of the user's meals [13]. For example, O'Loughlin et al. [14] examine the feasibility of utilizing the Microsoft SenseCam [15] (i.e., a wearable camera) to estimate the dietary energy intake within various sporting populations. However, these approaches may raise some privacy concerns due to the fact that camera could capture the user's personal sensitive information such as social relationships (i.e., eating with whom) and location privacy (i.e., where).

Recently, some wearable device based approaches have been proposed to detect the user's eating periods by leveraging the embedded sensors (e.g., microphones and motion sensors). Sazonov et al. [7] develop a system utilizing the piezoelectric sensor attached to the ear to detect the chewing and swallowing. Similarly, Bedri et al. [16] design an eating episode detection system by utilizing a dedicated ear-worn device, which is equipped with an inertial sensor behind the ear to detect people's dietary motions. Rather than the ear-worn sensor, Thomaz et al. [8] use the accelerometer on a smartwatch to infer eating moments to capture the user's hand motions during dietary period. Along this direction, Zhang et al. [17] propose a dedicated wearable device using wireless accelerometers attached on both wrists of users to detect the eating/drinking activities based on the three-dimensional kinematics movement model. Unfortunately, these wearable-based methods requiring the user to equip with dedicated hardware platforms during eating, which are obtrusive to users and also shows the limitation of their deployments in the practical scenarios.

Our work is different in that we propose a low user-effort dietary moments recognition system by leveraging the WiFi signals extracted from the user smartphone, which is a pervasive mobile device. Our system is low-cost and easy-to-use without additional dedicated devices or professional installations. Specifically, the proposed system could detect the eating episode on a daily life, including the starting/ending time of each meal, which provides an automatic solution to track the user's dietary schedule. Moreover, the system could identify the utensils held by the participants (e.g., folk and spoon) during the intake period and further segment the dietary moments into detailed eating episodes according to different utensils. Based on the comprehensive dietary information, it shows the potential to further infer how and what the users eat and measure the dietary behaviors of users.

3   System and Methodology

3.1   System Overview

The main goal of our work is to let user simply place his/her smartphone on the dinning table to achieve automatic fine-grained eating moment monitoring.

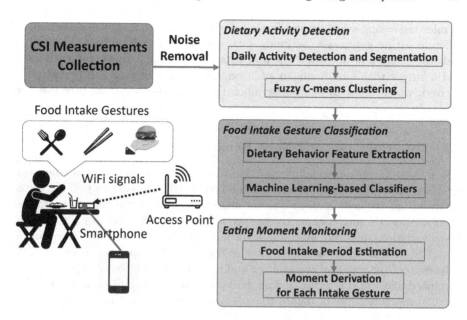

Fig. 1. Overview of the proposed system for eating moment monitoring.

The basic idea is to recognize the dietary moments by extracting the unique physiological and behavioral characteristics inherited from food intake gestures by leveraging the readily available WiFi signals. As illustrated in Fig. 1, the system takes the CSI measurements extracted from the personal mobile devices (i.e., smartphones) as the input. To mitigate the ambient noises and reduce the influence of wireless interference, we apply *Noise Removal* techniques to remove the outliers of CSI raw data and reduce the high and low frequency noises using a bandpass filter. Next, our system performs *Dietary Activity Detection* to distinguish the relative eating activities from many other daily human activities (e.g, walking, reading, talking) in the environment. Specifically, we examine the moving variance and accumulated short time energy (STE) of the calibrated CSI data to obtain the segments containing the user's daily activities. We then develop the *Fuzzy C-means Clustering* method to recognize the dietary activities in a cluster and differentiating them from non-eating activities based on calculating the Euclidean distance between eating cluster center and the test activity. To further identify the specific food intake gestures (i.e., eating with fork, spoon, knife, chopsticks and bare hands) of the user, the system extracts unique features from both time and frequency domains to capture the inherent physiological and behavioral characteristics of user's motions. Base on the extracted features, we perform *Food Intake Gesture Classification* to recognize the user's different eating gestures. We test several different machine learning classifiers including Random Forest (RF), Naive Bayes (NB), K Nearest Neighbors (KNN), Discriminant Analysis Classifier (DAC), respectively. The last component *Eating Moment Estimation* estimates the food intake period of the user to infer the eating schedule and further divide the eating moments according to different eating gestures to estimate eating episode of each gesture. The eating gestures reflect how and what the user eats, for example eating steak with knife and a burger with bare hand. In addition, the number of each eating gesture is derived, which helps to know how much the user eats as well as how fast the user eats.

3.2 Data Collection and Noise Removal

CSI measurements are readily available from some commodity WiFi network interface controller (NIC) such as the Intel 5300 NIC. In order to perform automatic eating moment monitoring, we utilize the CSI measurements extracted from a subject's smartphone, to capture the minute differences of the channel state variations induced by a subject's food intake gestures. The intuition is that CSI measurement describes how a WiFi signal propagates over multiple subcarriers from a pair of transmitter and receiver. In addition, it represents the combined effect of scattering, fading, and power decay with distances. Specially, the CSI measurements in regard to each subcarrier can be denoted as:

$$H_k = |H_k| e^{j \angle H_k}, \tag{1}$$

where $|H_k|$ and $\angle H_k$ describe the corresponding amplitude and phase. They represent the signal interference impacted by the human body movements, including absorption, reflection and refraction by food intake gestures. However, a subject's eating activity is very complicated since people perform different ways using their arm to take food from plate to mouth. Besides, the intake process may involve different utensils (i.e., spoon, fork, knife, and chopsticks), increasing the difficulty to perform fine-grained eating recognition. In that case, we need to extract more information based on the raw CSI measurements to provide an accurate description of the wireless signals.

Since the existing of ambient noises in daily dining environments, the WiFi signals also suffer from signal scattering and wireless interference. To mitigate the ambient noises on the CSI measurements, our system first applies a band-pass filter to remove the noises of high-frequency and low-frequency to ensure the reliability of WIFI signals. According to our observations the frequency of relative environment noises usually present in a fixed frequency range, we thus utilize an empirical threshold to remove the ambient noises.

3.3 Dietary Activity Detection

Daily Activity Detection and Segmentation. After removing the irrelevant ambient noises, we perform daily activity detection and segmentation on the CSI measurements that mapping the wireless signal with the people's daily activities. Inspired by experiment observations, we find that human activities (i.e., walking, standing) involved the body movements lead to some vibrations on the CSI raw data. However, the variances caused by body movements usually present as a

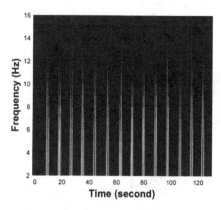

Fig. 2. Accumulated power spectral density of CSI in frequency domain.

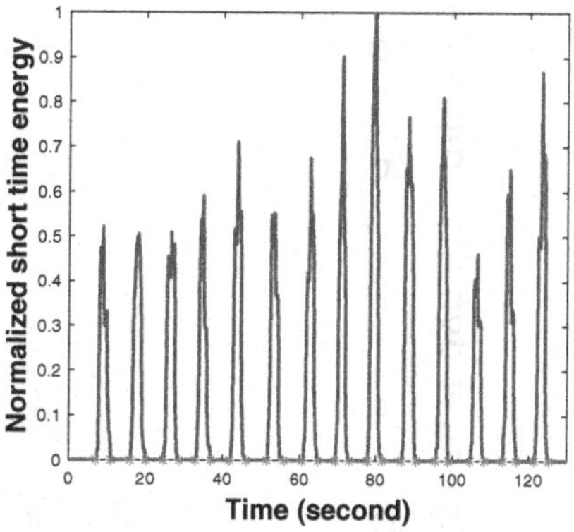

Fig. 3. Illustration of the STE-based activity detection and segmentation.

non-obvious pattern and hard to be detected. Moreover, dietary activities (e.g., using fork to bring food from dining table to mouth) usually involved minute scale body movements than walking activities, which increases the difficulty of detection. To enlarge the variances in original CSI measurements, we thus adopt a spectrogram-based approach to calculate the short time energy (STE) upon CSI amplitude's moving variance to detect human activity. As shown in Fig. 2, we derive the STE by calculating the integration of power spectral density along the frequency domain. Additionally, STE approach is more sensitive to human body movements by reconstructing the minute motions within a sliding window, which also enlarges the variances in frequency domain upon CSI measurements. We calculate STE by the following formula:

$$STE(\delta) = \sum_{i=1}^{I}[PSD(\delta)W(\delta + i)]^2, \tag{2}$$

where $PSD(\delta)$ represents the power spectral density function, $W(\delta)$ denotes the window function and I is the length of the sliding window. Figure 3 shows the segments of human activities (i.e., use bare hands to bring food to mouth). It is obvious that STE demonstrated as great values when the dietary activity occurs. Moreover, we found there are some peaks always locate at the center of the activity duration. Inspired by this, we define the two adjacent zero points to segment the corresponding human activities.

Fuzzy C-means Clustering. After detecting all of the daily activities from users, we apply an unsupervised clustering method to further differentiate the related dietary activities from the human daily activities. The basic idea is the dietary activities are defined as the arm and hand gestures involved in bringing food to the mouth from a dining table, which are tiny movements and similar to each others. However, other daily activities such as walking or standing involved

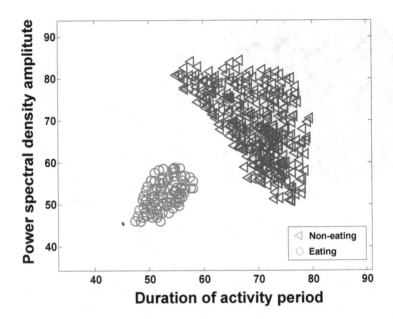

Fig. 4. Fuzzy C-Means cluster results of eating activity and non-eating activity.

large body movements (e.g., swing arms, bending over) might conduct more intensive vibrations in the frequency domain of CSI measurements. Motivated by this, we then examine to use the Fuzzy C-Means Clustering (FCM) approach to assort the data into two clusters based on two-dimensional features including the PSD Amplitude and corresponding frequency of these activities. The FCM-based Clustering could be described as:

$$\Upsilon_m = \sum_{i=1}^{A}\sum_{j=1}^{N} \mu_{ij}^m \|A_i - C_j\|^2, \tag{3}$$

where A denotes the number of human activity segments, N is the number of clusters, m denotes the fuzzy partition matrix exponent of controlling the degree of fuzzy overlap, A_i represents the ith activity segments, C_j denotes the center of the jth cluster, μ_{ij} represents the degree of membership of A_i in the jth cluster.

In order to understand the distribution of participants dietary activities and other daily activities, we first ran a formative study with 2 participants to perform 10 different motions in lab environment. Participants were requested to eat a variety of foods including chips, pizza, bread and noodles with their bare hands, forks, chopsticks. Moreover, we ask participant to perform some non-eating activity including walking, standing, sitting, talking, reading, typing, stretching, respectively. Figure 4 shows the clustering results regarding eating activities and non-eating activities. We note that the proposed approach could successful differentiate the activities into two clusters. In addition, we observe the eating activities are mainly gathered in the lower range of duration period

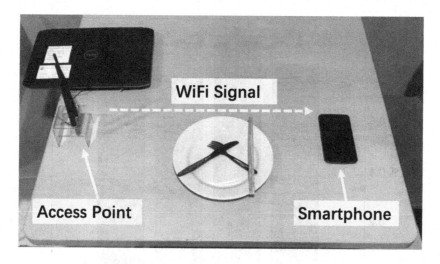

Fig. 5. Illustration of our experimental setting.

than non-dietary activities are located in the higher range. This is because during the ingestion period, participants keep bringing food to mouth in a repetitive manner, and the eating motions performed by participants usually take faster than other non-dietary activities such as the walking. Based on the differentiate results, we thus can utilize the derived dietary activities to further process fine-grained classification in terms of the utensils held by users.

3.4 Food Intake Gesture Classification

In our system, recognizing various food intake gesture is essential for deriving find-grained statistic information and further detecting eating moments. Among this section, we adopt various machine learning classifiers to identify different eating gestures. We first extract a series of features both from time and frequency domains from thirty subcarriers and then derive two-dimensional vectors as the inputs of multiple classifiers. In order to motivate the suitability of the proposed method with different machine learning algorithm, we apply four kinds of typical machine learning methods (i.e., Random Forest (RF), Naive Bayes (NB), K Nearest Neighbors (KNN), and Discriminant Analysis Classifier (DAC)) to recognize various eating gestures according to the utensils held by the user, including spoon, fork, fork&knife, hand and chopsticks. The machine learning algorithms are implemented based on the Statistics and Machine Learning Toolbox of Matlab R2019a. We further evaluate the performance of the four traditional classifiers and discuss the results in Sect. 4.2.

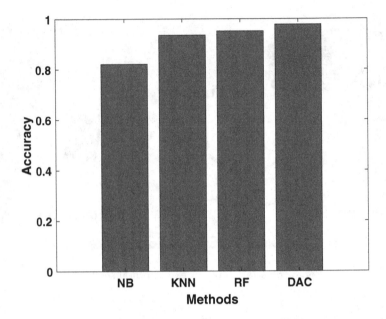

Fig. 6. Comparison of performance among four kinds of machine learning classifiers for food intake gestures identification.

3.5 Eating Moment Monitoring

Our intuition of monitoring the eating moment for users is to further estimate the accurate ingestion duration between the interval of each separate food intake gestures. Study [18] shows that the eating speed is positively associated with body weight-gain, indicating that the fast eating speed might increase the risk of overweight and obesity. Thus, it is essential to obtain the fine-grained ingestion period statistics (e.g., the duration time for participants to eat with fork, spoon or chopsticks) to further elaborate and evaluate the user's eating behaviors. Given that intuition, we adopt the intake gesture density derivation method to infer the eating moment based on calculating the density of detection food intake gestures when applying a sliding window in a specific eating period length. To compare the prediction estimated dietary duration with the ground truth, we evaluate the detailed results of eating moment monitoring in Sect. 4.3.

4   Performance Evaluation

4.1 Experimental Methodology

As shown in Fig. 5, we implement our system with a pair of WiFi-enabled devices, including a smartphone and a laptop. Our system aims to imitate the real scenario when people are eating and placing their smartphones on the dining table. In the system, user's smartphone will send WiFi signals to the access point

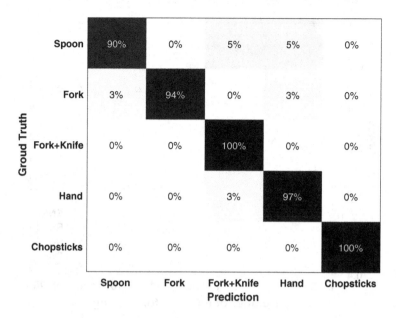

Fig. 7. Confusion matrix of food intake gestures classification.

and sense different eating activities. To conduct experiments, we use a Nexus 6 smartphone powered by a 2.7 GHz quad-core Snapdragon 805 processor with 3 GB of RAM as the transmitter. For the receiver, we use a Dell E6430 equipped with Intel 5300 802.11n WiFi wireless card and 6dBi rubber ducky external omni-directional antennas for extracting CSI readings [19]. The laptop which serves as the access point is configured to run in the netlink mode. Internet Control Message Protocol (ICMP) echo is sent from the laptop and replied by the smartphone to collect the CSI data [20]. In total, 10 volunteers are recruited as the subjects to take part in the experiments and finally we collect 400 min length data for eating episode. Moreover, the distance between the laptop and the smartphone is 80 cm. Unless mentioned otherwise, half of the collection data is used for training and the rest for testing.

4.2 Performance of Food Intake Gesture Classification

We first compare the performance of food intake gesture classification under four typical machine learning classifiers including Random Forest (RF), Naive Bayes (NB), K Nearest Neighbors (KNN), and Discriminant Analysis Classifier (DAC). The parameters of each classifier are tuned to achieve the best performance. As shown in Fig. 6, for eating gesture recognition, all the classifiers achieve average accuracy over 80%, indicating that our model could perform well with various classifiers. Specifically, NB, KNN, RF and DAC have average accuracy of 82.1%, 93.6%, 95.2%, 97.8%, respectively. We observe that DAC achieves the best eating gesture identification results. For each eating gesture as depicted in Fig. 7,

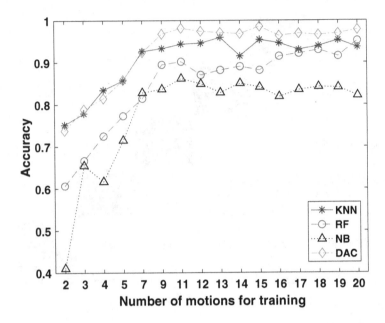

Fig. 8. The impact of training size on the eating gesture recognition.

the DAC achieves average accuracy of 90%, 94%, 100%, 97% and 100% for five eating gestures (i.e., spoon, fork, fork&knife, hand, chopsticks). The experimental results show that various eating gestures can all be well recognized by the proposed system. Furthermore, we evaluate the impact of different training sizes on the eating gesture recognition. Figure 8 shows that our system could achieve over 80% accuracy under different training sizes and even 7 eating motions is sufficient to produce over 80% accuracy, which further confirms the effectiveness of our system.

4.3   Performance of Eating Moment Monitoring

Coarse Eating Moment Recognition. To determine the starting point and the ending point of eating moment, we first evaluate our system performance on distinguishing eating activities from non-eating activities. Figure 9 provides a detailed picture of the FCM-based cluster performance with different m value, where m denotes the fuzzy partition matrix exponent of controlling the degree of fuzzy overlap. As shown in the figure, our system achieves an accuracy over 90% when m is over 1.6. We also note that our system achieves 95% accuracy on eating and non-eating activity recognition given an m value of 2.4. This is because m represents the average coefficient related to the distribution clustering results and enlarging value of m could convey more controlling degree to maximize the distances between different clusters and minimize the inner distance of clusters regarding the eating activities and non-eating activities.

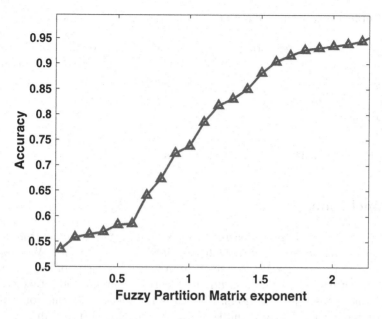

Fig. 9. The performance of dietary activity extraction under various fuzzy partition matrix exponent of FCM clustering.

Intake Gesture Moment Estimation. Then we evaluate the performance of dietary moment recognition for different food intake gestures. In our experiments, each participant is requested to eat a variety of foods with five kinds of gestures for multiple times. In particular, each gesture will be repeated for 40 times and we collected 200 eating activities for each person in total. As shown in Table 1, the average estimated time duration of using spoon, fork, fork&knife, hand, and chopsticks are 5 m 43 s, 5 m 34 s, 7 m 57 s, 6 m 37 s, 6 m 34 s respectively. While the corresponding ground truths are 5 m 20 s, 5 m 52 s, 8 m 11 s, 5 m 53 s, 6 m 18 s respectively. And the ground truths are measured and verified by camera based method during the experiment. We find that the estimated error of five intake gestures are 23 s, 18 s, 14 s, 44 s, and 16 s. In particular, the average duration error of one single eating gesture is within 1.1 s. Through analyzing the time duration of each eating gesture, we can have a comprehensive understanding of the dietary moment for each user. Based on the derived fine-grained dietary statistics, it is easy to infer other high-level information such as the estimation of calories intake, analysis of nutritional balance. In addition, the detailed dietary information can also be used to assist various health related problems such as cardiovascular diseases, diabetes, stomach cancers.

Table 1. The average duration of each eating gesture across all users.

Eating gesture	Estimated eating moment	Ground truth	Estimated error	Average estimation error for each gesture
Spoon	5 m 43 s	5 m 20 s	23 s	0.58 s
Fork	5 m 34 s	5 m 52 s	18 s	0.45 s
Fork&Knife	7 m 57 s	8 m 11 s	14 s	0.35 s
Hand	6 m 37 s	5 m 53 s	44 s	1.1 s
Chopsticks	6 m 34 s	6 m 18 s	16 s	0.4 s

5   Conclusion

In this paper, we explore the feasibility of leveraging WiFi signals from smartphones to automatically monitor the fine-grained eating moments. We show that the channel state information extracted from a user's smartphone could be utilized to detect eating activity and further identify different food intake gestures based on the utensils held by users. The statistical dietary information could be used to interpret the detailed intake duration and utensil types during eating period. It also shows the potential to provide the comprehensive understanding with users regarding their eating behaviors and help them to build a healthy dietary pattern. We develop a device-free system, which first differentiates eating activities from non-eating activities based on a fuzzy c-means clustering method. We then utilize the learning-based methods to classify the user's food intake gestures according to the utensils held by the user with four different classifiers (i.e., Random Forest, Naive Bayes, K Nearest Neighbors and Discriminant Analysis Classier). Furthermore, we derive the food intake duration and further estimate the eating moments for each food intake gesture. Extensive experimental results with 10 subjects over 400-min eating period show that our system can recognize the user's food intake gestures with up to 97.8% accuracy and estimate the dietary moments within 1.1-s error.

Acknowledgment. This work was supported by the National Science Foundation Grant CNS-1826647.

References

1. Mokdad, A.H., et al.: Prevalence of obesity, diabetes, and obesity-related health risk factors, 2001. JAMA **289**(1), 76–79 (2003)
2. World Health Organization: What are the health consequences of being overweight? https://www.who.int/features/qa/49/en//. Accessed 17 Apr 2019
3. World Health Organization: Infobase page for illustrating overweight & obesity diseases. https://www.who.int/news-room/fact-sheets/detail/obesity-and-overweight/. Accessed 17 Apr 2019
4. Loewy, J.: My macros+—diet and calories. https://itunes.apple.com/us/app/my-macros-diet-calories/id475249619/. Accessed 21 Apr 2019

5. Feel great about what you ate (2019). https://youate.com/
6. Hill, R., Davies, P.: The validity of self-reported energy intake as determined using the doubly labelled water technique. Br. J. Nutr. **85**(4), 415–430 (2001)
7. Sazonov, E., et al.: Non-invasive monitoring of chewing and swallowing for objective quantification of ingestive behavior. Physiol. Meas. **29**(5), 525 (2008)
8. Thomaz, E., Essa, I., Abowd, G.D.: A practical approach for recognizing eating moments with wrist-mounted inertial sensing. In: Proceedings of the 2015 ACM International Joint Conference on Pervasive and Ubiquitous Computing, pp. 1029–1040. ACM (2015)
9. Guo, X., Liu, J., Shi, C., Liu, H., Chen, Y., Chuah, M.C.: Device-free personalized fitness assistant using WiFi. Proc. ACM Interact. Mob. Wearable Ubiquit. Technol. **2**(4), 165 (2018)
10. Liu, J., Wang, Y., Chen, Y., Yang, J., Chen, X., Cheng, J.: Tracking vital signs during sleep leveraging off-the-shelf WiFi. In: Proceedings of the 16th ACM International Symposium on Mobile Ad Hoc Networking and Computing (ACM MobiHoc), pp. 267–276 (2015)
11. Wang, Y., Liu, J., Chen, Y., Gruteser, M., Yang, J., Liu, H.: E-eyes: device-free location-oriented activity identification using fine-grained WiFi signatures. In: Proceedings of the 20th Annual International Conference on Mobile Computing and Networking, pp. 617–628. ACM (2014)
12. Willett, W.: Nutritional Epidemiology, vol. 40. Oxford University Press, Oxford (2012)
13. Sun, M., et al.: A wearable electronic system for objective dietary assessment. J. Am. Diet. Assoc. **110**(1), 45–47 (2010)
14. O'Loughlin, G., et al.: Using a wearable camera to increase the accuracy of dietary analysis. Am. J. Prev. Med. **44**(3), 297–301 (2013)
15. Hodges, S., et al.: SenseCam: a retrospective memory aid. In: Dourish, P., Friday, A. (eds.) UbiComp 2006. LNCS, vol. 4206, pp. 177–193. Springer, Heidelberg (2006). https://doi.org/10.1007/11853565_11
16. Bedri, A., et al.: EarBit: using wearable sensors to detect eating episodes in unconstrained environments. Proc. ACM Interact. Mob. Wearable Ubiquit. Technol. **1**(3), 37 (2017)
17. Zhang, S., Ang, M., Xiao, W., Tham, C.K.: Detection of activities by wireless sensors for daily life surveillance: eating and drinking. Sensors **9**(3), 1499–1517 (2009)
18. Ohkuma, T., Hirakawa, Y., Nakamura, U., Kiyohara, Y., Kitazono, T., Ninomiya, T.: Association between eating rate and obesity: a systematic review and meta-analysis. Int. J. Obes. **39**(11), 1589 (2015)
19. Halperin, D., Hu, W., Sheth, A., Wetherall, D.: Tool release: gathering 802.11 n traces with channel state information. ACM SIGCOMM Comput. Commun. Rev. **41**(1), 53–53 (2011)
20. Li, M., et al.: When CSI meets public WiFi: inferring your mobile phone password via WiFi signals. In: Proceedings of the 2016 ACM SIGSAC Conference on Computer and Communications Security, pp. 1068–1079. ACM (2016)

SocialBike: Quantified-Self Data as Social Cue in Physical Activity

Nan Yang[1(✉)], Gerbrand van Hout[2], Loe Feijs[1], Wei Chen[3],
and Jun Hu[1]

[1] Department of Industrial Design, Eindhoven University of Technology,
5600 MB Eindhoven, The Netherlands
{n.yang,l.m.g.feijs,j.hu}@tue.nl
[2] Obesity Centre, Catharina Hospital, 5623 EJ Eindhoven, The Netherlands
info@drvanhout.nl
[3] Department of Electronic Engineering, Fudan University,
Shanghai 200433, China
w_chen@fudan.edu.cn

Abstract. Quantified-self application is widely used in sports and health management; the type and amount of data that can be fed back to the user are growing rapidly. However, only a few studies discussed the social attributes of quantified-self data, especially in the context of cycling. In this study, we present "SocialBike," a digital augmented bicycle that aims to increase cyclists' motivation and social relatedness in physical activity by showing their quantified-self data to each other. To evaluate the concept through a rigorous control experiment, we built a cycling simulation system to simulate a realistic cycling experience with SocialBike. A within-subjects experiment was conducted through the cycling simulation system with 20 participants. Quantitative data were collected with the Intrinsic Motivation Inventory (IMI) and data recorded by the simulation system; qualitative data were collected through user interviews. The result showed that SocialBike increase cyclists' intrinsic motivation, perceived competence, and social relatedness in physical activity.

Keywords: Social interaction · Quantified-self · Personal informatics · Motivation · Physical activity · Health

1 Introduction

Health tracking devices and applications have become increasingly ubiquitous. By accurately monitoring and systematically recording personal information, these applications help users manage their exercise, diet, or sleep. In addition to providing feedback to individual users, some applications offer social sharing capabilities (Fitbit, Nike+, Garmin, etc.), including in-app data sharing and data sharing to other social networks such as Facebook, Twitter, and Instagram. Epstein et al. [1] summarized six reasons why people share their personal informatics data: request for information, desire for emotional support, seeking motivation or accountability from the audience, motivating or informing the sharing audience, impression management.

N. M. Garcia et al. (Eds.): HealthyIoT 2019, LNICST 314, pp. 92–107, 2020.

However, in this form of remote personal data sharing, there are gaps in time and space between the sharer and sharing audience. For instance, people can only share their exercise history after the actual exercise. When the sharing audience sees this information, their psychological and physiological state could be completely different from the sharer. These gaps create obstacles to the establishment of empathy and social connection between the sharer and the sharing audience. In face-to-face social interaction, people can use both verbal and non-verbal cues [2, 3] to communicate with each other, but digital information is hard to be used to facilitate communication, especially in the context of physical activity.

We tried to provide a channel for sharing digital information in a face-to-face social context; in other words, incorporate a digital communication layer into the physical world. Therefore, in this paper, we present SocialBike, a digital augmented bicycle that allows users to show their selected quantified-self data to other cyclists nearby. An experiment was conducted through a cycling simulation system with 20 participants. We examined the effect of SocialBike on increasing cyclists' motivation and social relatedness in physical activity.

2 Related Work

2.1 Quantified-Self Data in Social Contexts

Quantified-self data can be used to support health management or exercise. In addition to applications at the individual level, some studies have also explored the social application of quantified-self data. Epstein et al. [1] presented a design framework for social sharing in personal informatics. Ivanov et al. [4] explored factors that impact sharing health-tracking records; they investigated the influence of health motivation, perceived health status, the severity of health, and age on the sharing of self-tracked information. HeartLink [5] is an application that collects real-time personal biometric data in sports events and broadcasts this data online. "Jogging over a Distance" [6] is a system use spatialized audio based on heart rate to support runners in a different country running together.

Research on sharing quantified-self data is not limited to remote sharing via social networks or mobile applications. Some research applies quantified-self data to face-to-face social context. "Social Fabric Fitness" [7] is a wearable E-Textile display designed to support group running, it provides a shared screen on the back of the wearer's shirt, displaying information such as heart rate and pace. Walmink et al. [8] presented a bicycle helmet that can display heart rate to support social exertion experience. "Race by Hearts" [9] is a mobile application that enables competition based on heart rate data sharing between users in real-time.

2.2 Digitally Enhanced Face-to-Face Social Expression

In addition to quantified-self data, some other innovative digital forms are also applied by researchers to enhance face-to-face social expression. Beilharz et al. [10] presented a wearable device that uses physical analog visualization and digital sonification to convey feedback about the wearer's activity and environment. Walmink et al. [11] explored interaction opportunities around helmet design; they presented the concept of LumaHelm that turns the helmet into a display for communication, expression, and play.

Fluxa [12] is a wearable device that exploits body movements; it uses persistence of vision (POV) effect to generate mid-air social displays. Lighting effects were also widely used in textile design [13–15] and wearable devices [16–19] to enrich the wearer's social expression.

Some research tried to expand the social attributes of existing personal electronics devices, such as laptops [20] and smartwatches [21].

3   Design and Implementation

3.1   Design of SocialBike

SocialBike is a digital augmented bicycle designed to increase cyclists' motivation and social relatedness in physical activity. It allows users to show their selected quantified-self data to other cyclists nearby.

SocialBike consists of a mobile app based on Google Fit API [22] and an on-bike display. With the Google Fit platform, the mobile apps can get data from any health tracking devices that are compatible with Google Fit API (Fig. 1) [23]. In the mobile app, users can select the type and form of quantified-self data they want to display and send it to the on-bike display (Fig. 2).

The data type that SocialBike can display includes both real-time data such as heart rate and speed, as well as historical data over time, such as total distance, total steps, and total calorie consumption.

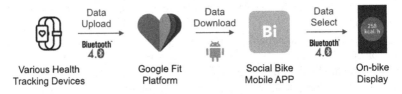

Fig. 1. Schematic of SocialBike's technical system.

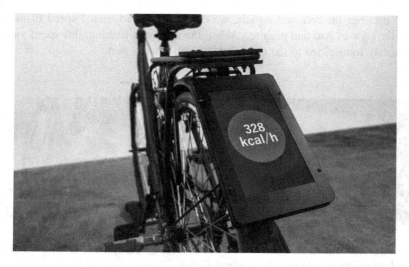

Fig. 2. Prototype of SocialBike's on-bike display.

3.2 Cycling Simulation System

In order to conduct rigorous control experiments, a cycling simulation system was built to simulate a realistic riding experience with SocialBike. The hardware composition of the system is shown in Fig. 3.

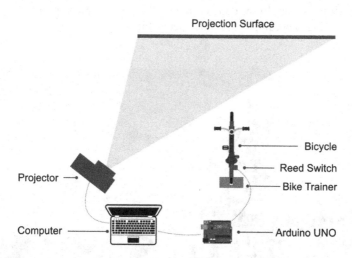

Fig. 3. Schematic of the cycling simulation system (top view).

A reed switch was mounted on the bike frame near the rear wheel, and a magnet was clamped to the spokes of the rear wheel (Fig. 4). Each time the rear wheel turns 360 degrees, the reed switch sends a signal to the Arduino Uno board. Based on the interval between the received signals, we calculated the rotational speed of the rear wheels through an Arduino program. When the system is running, this speed value is continuously transmitted to the computer through a serial port.

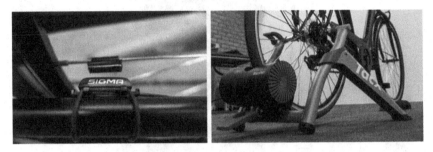

Fig. 4. The reed switch and magnet used to detect the rotational speed of the bike wheel (left) and the bike trainer used to provide resistance (right).

In addition, a bike trainer is used to simulate the friction of the bike wheel rolling on the real ground (Fig. 4).

The software part of the cycling simulation system was built with Unity 3D and running on a computer. The simulated scene in the program will be projected on a large surface in front of the bike. When the computer receives the rational speed value from a serial port, the simulation program will convert it to line speed base on the diameter of the bicycle wheel. When the system is running, the user's viewpoint in the simulation program is moving according to the line speed (Fig. 5).

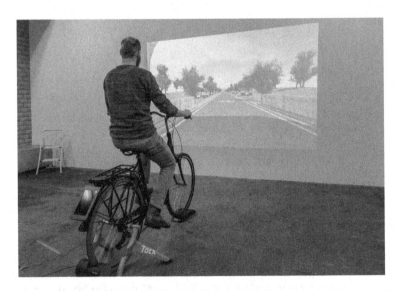

Fig. 5. Cycling simulation system in test.

Since the study was conducted in the Netherlands, and all participants we recruited lived in the Netherlands. Therefore, in the scenario design of the simulation program, we used the elements of the Dutch bicycle lane to make the scene as close as possible to the local appearance (Fig. 6).

In the simulated scenario, the user will see other virtual cyclists riding their own SocialBike. The data displayed on virtual cyclists' bikes also change in real-time based on their riding speed (Fig. 6).

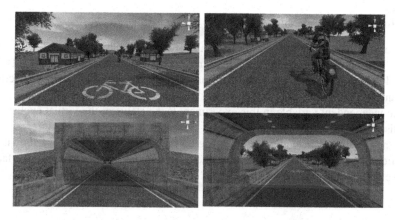

Fig. 6. Screenshots of different scenes in the simulation program.

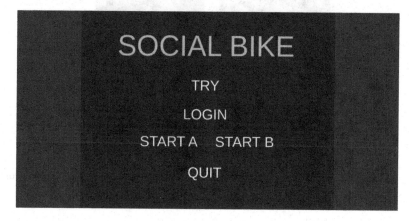

Fig. 7. Start menu of the simulation program.

Since the cycling simulation system is designed for experimentation, it has the ability to record experimental data. Participants' basic information can be entered into the system through the start menu (Fig. 7). At the end of each experiment, the system automatically generates a log file in .csv format. The log file contains all data related to participant's riding behavior in the experiment, such as position, speed, and distance to the virtual cyclist [24].

4   Evaluation

4.1   Subjects

Twenty participants (10 females, 10 males, age range: 27–41 years) participated in the study through informed consent procedures. All participants had experience in riding an ordinary bicycle. Each participant was compensated with 5 euros for their participation.

4.2   Independent Variable

In this experiment, we evaluated the influence of other people's quantified-self data on participants' behavior and mental state. Therefore, the bicycle that the participants were riding do not display their own data, but they can see the data of the virtual cyclist in the simulated scenario.

The independent variable in this experiment is the status of the virtual cyclist's on-bike display in the simulation program.

In the experiment scenario, the interface on the virtual cyclist's bike is showing an animation of his calorie consumption per hour. In the control scenario, the interface is inactive and shows a black screen (Fig. 8).

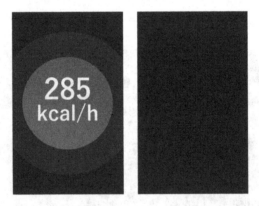

Fig. 8. The status of the independent variable in the experiment scenario (left) and the control scenario (right).

4.3   Measurements

The Intrinsic Motivation Inventory (IMI) [25] was used to evaluate the effect of the independent variable on participants' intrinsic motivation for physical activity and social relatedness with other cyclists. According to the instruction of the inventory, there are three questions in subscale "Value/Usefulness" needs to be completed by the researcher base on the questions they are addressing [25]. Therefore, we used "encouraging me to do more physical activity" to complete these three questions.

Participant's riding behavior data was automatically recorded by the simulation system. From the log files generated by the system, we extracted "the total time participant stays with the virtual cyclist within 5 m" as an indicator of social relatedness.

A semi-structured interview was conducted at the end of each experiment. The result of the interview was used to support the quantitative data and provide insights for further research.

4.4   Setup

The experiment was conducted in a laboratory with the cycling simulation system (Fig. 3). The simulated scenario was projected on a large surface in front of the bicycle. The size of the projected area is 291 cm wide and 188 cm high. The distance from the bicycle's front wheel to the projection surface is 160 cm (Fig. 9). All of these dimensions were designed to ensure that the simulated scenario showed to the participant was closest to the real-world perspective. The computer, projector, sensor, and all other devices used in the experiment were placed outside the subject's field of view.

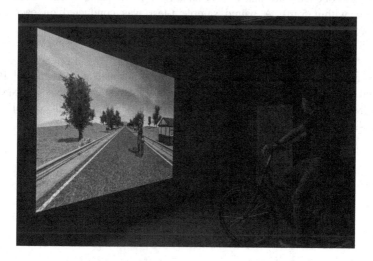

Fig. 9. The experiment setup of SocialBike.

4.5   Procedure

Participants were randomly divided into two groups, group 1 and group 2. Before the formal experiment begins, we gave each participant a brief instruction about the experiment and let them read and sign the consent form. Then participants were invited to ride on the simulator with a free-riding mode for 2 min with the purpose of getting familiar with the riding simulation system.

The formal riding experiment has two sessions. In session A, each participant was introduced to the concept of SocialBike and asked to ride on the experiment scenario for 5 min. After that, they were asked to complete an IMI questionnaire [25] according to their experience. In session B, the participant was asked to ride on the control scenario for 5 min and complete an IMI questionnaire too.

In order to eliminate the influence of the order, participants in group 1 were asked to carry out session A before session B, participants in group 2 were asked to carry out session B before session A. Each participant had a 10-min break between the two sessions. At the end of each experiment, a semi-structured interview was conducted with the participant. Each interview took about ten minutes, and the interview was audio-recorded and transcribed by the researcher.

5 Result

5.1 Quantitative Result

Eight types of quantitative data were collected, including seven subscales in the Intrinsic Motivation Inventory (IMI) (Interest/Enjoyment, Perceived Competence, Effort/Importance, Pressure/Tension, Perceived Choice, Value/Usefulness, Relatedness) [25], and one indicator that we extracted from participants' cycling behavior data (Total time within 5 m). A paired sample t-test was conducted on each type of quantitative data to evaluate the effect of SocialBike.

5.1.1 Interest/Enjoyment

This subscale is considered the self-report measure of intrinsic motivation [25]. Base on the paired sample t-test, participants' feeling of interest/enjoyment in experiment scenario (Mean = 5.087 SD = 0.846) was significantly higher than in control scenario (Mean = 4.171 SD = 1.184), t(19) = 3.180, p = 0.005, r = 0.232 (Fig. 10).

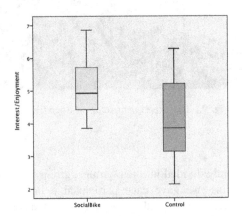

Fig. 10. The result of Interest/Enjoyment (ranges from 1–7).

5.1.2   Perceived Competence

Participants' perceived competence level in experiment scenario (Mean = 5.125, SD = 0.825) was significantly higher than in control scenario (Mean = 4.675, SD = 0.933), t(19) = 2.862, p = 0.010, r = 0.686 (Fig. 11).

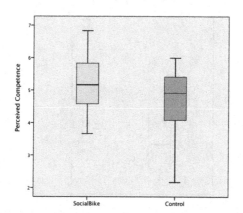

Fig. 11. The result of Perceived Competence (ranges from 1–7).

5.1.3   Effort/Importance

As regards the effort/importance, there was no significant difference between the result in experiment scenario (Mean = 3.920, SD = 0.916) and in control scenario (Mean = 3.750, SD = 0.929), t(19) = 0.923, p = 0.368, r = 0.601 (Fig. 12).

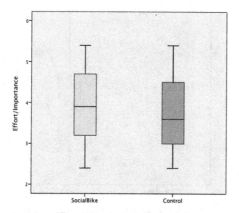

Fig. 12. The result of Effort/Importance (ranges from 1–7).

5.1.4   Pressure/Tension

Participants' feeling of pressure/tension had no significant difference in experiment scenario (Mean = 2.230, SD = 1.001) and in control scenario (Mean = 2.400, SD = 0.902), t(19) = −1.116, p = 0.278, r = 0.748 (Fig. 13).

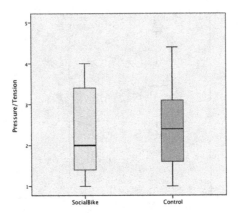

Fig. 13. The result of Pressure/Tension (ranges from 1–7).

5.1.5   Perceived Choice

Participants' perceived choice level had no significant difference in experiment scenario (Mean = 5.185, SD = 0.966) and in control scenario (Mean = 4.757, SD = 1.142), t(19) = 1.949, p = 0.066, r = 0.576 (Fig. 14).

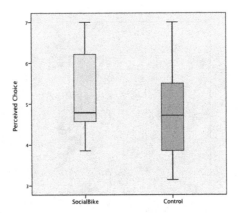

Fig. 14. The result of Perceived Choice (ranges from 1–7).

5.1.6   Value/Usefulness

Value/usefulness perceived by participants in experiment scenario (Mean = 5.643, SD = 0.971) was significantly higher than in control scenario (Mean = 4.743, SD = 1.282), t(19) = 3.846, p = 0.001, r = 0.603 (Fig. 15).

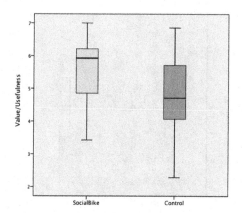

Fig. 15. The result of Value/Usefulness (ranges from 1–7).

5.1.7   Relatedness

Participants felt significantly stronger relatedness with other cyclist in experiment scenario (Mean = 4.481, SD = 1.209) than in control scenario (Mean = 3.519, SD = 1.033), t(19) = 3.115, p = 0.006, r = 0.248 (Fig. 16).

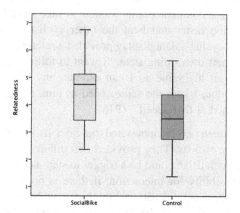

Fig. 16. The result of Relatedness (ranges from 1–7).

5.1.8 Total Time Within 5 m

The total time that participants keep within 5 m with the virtual cyclist in experiment scenario (Mean = 126.200, SD = 85.189) is significantly longer than in control scenario (Mean = 72.050, SD = 61.381), t(19) = 3.226, p = 0.004, r = 0.515 (Fig. 17).

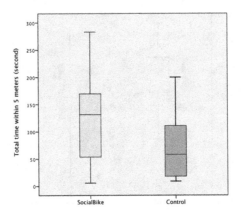

Fig. 17. The result of Total time within 5 m (ranges from 0–300).

5.2 Result of Interview

Motivation. Eighteen participants (out of 20) reported that SocialBike increased their motivation for cycling. Eight participants stated that they felt a competitive relationship with the virtual cyclist during the experiment. "With this data, I paid more attention to him. I regarded him as a competitor and wanted to take over him." (P20). "I was motivated. I tried to ride faster and beat the other cyclist." (P1). Ten participants reported that the virtual cyclist's data display provided a reference for them so that they can better understand their own riding state. "I want to follow this person; on the one hand, I am curious about his value so I can estimate my own value." (P5). "I am concerned about this value, I kept the same speed as him, so I can know how many calories will be consumed at that speed." (P16).

Social Interaction. Sixteen participants stated that SocialBike Increased their desire to communicate with other cyclists. They provided two different explanations. 10 participants mentioned that SocialBike could be a trigger to start a conversation, for instance, "…it opens up the possibility for interaction, if there is no information, I don't feel connected with him, if there is information, I think it could be a starting point that I can cycle with him, or have a talk later." (P8) "Without this display, I wouldn't have a point to start talking to him." (P9). Six participants reported that they believe this person is willing to interact with others because he has actively shown his personal data. "He chose to show the information, means that he is a relatively open person; he wants to interact with others." (P10). "I saw that he showed some data; I felt a little closer to him. Showing this information will affect the sense of distance between him and me.

I think he showed a friendly intention, which may have an icebreaking effect." (P15). "He shared this information, meaning he is willing to communicate with others." (P20).

Data Display. Seventeen participants stated that real-time calorie consumption data is helpful for their cycling. However, 3 participants reported that they did not know the exact meaning of this value, and they preferred a more intuitive presentation of calorie consumption. "I need to know what is the meaning of that number, if I know that, it will be more motivating for me" (P7). "I do not know what 200 calories mean. If it can be converted into the corresponding food, I will have stronger motivation." (P2). We also asked each participant if SocialBike could display other data types, what they wanted to show on their own bike. "Speed" was mentioned by 8 participants, "heart rate" and "total distance" was mentioned by 3 participants, "cycling route" was mentioned by 2 participants. Other options such as "slope", "achievement", "badge", "emoji" were also mentioned.

6   Discussion

6.1   The Data Type and Display Form

In this experiment, the quantified-self data we used is calorie consumption per hour. Since SocialBike can collect and display various types of data, other data types could also be implemented and evaluated in a future iteration. The result of the interview shows that users prefer to display real-time quantified self-data during the ride. Compared to historical data over time, real-time data will change dynamically in a short period. Therefore, participants have less concern about privacy issues when showing their real-time data. In future iterations, we will prioritize the use of real-time data in the design process. In addition, when displaying quantified-self data during cycling, the strategy of data visualization should be simple and intuitive. It is not necessary to excessively pursue the accuracy of the data presented.

6.2   The Influence of Mutual Data Display

In this study, we focus on the influence of other people's quantified-self data on participants' behavior and mental state. However, in the full concept of SocailBike, the data display between cyclists is mutual. If participants have a clear awareness of the data they are presenting to others, then SocialBike may have a different impact on them. In order to evaluate this impact in future studies, a front interface could be provided to the user to let them compare their data with other cyclists' data. Considering the riding safety, the information displayed on the front interface should be simple, conspicuous, and does not take too much attention from the cyclist.

6.3   The Simulated Cycling Experience

The cycling simulation system allows us to perform rigorous control experiments in the laboratory. In the design of the cycling simulation system, we have considered the inertia, friction, light, and many other environmental factors. Although there are always some inevitable differences between the simulated scene and the real environment, we still find some space for improvement through this study. During the interview, many participants expressed satisfaction with the visual experience of the simulator. However, one participant stated that there was a lack of auditory experience during the ride. In order to make the user's riding experience more realistic in future iterations, the auditory experience can be introduced by adding ambient sound effects to the program.

7 Conclusion

In this study, we explored the opportunity of incorporating a digital communication channel into the context of social cycling. SocialBike was presented as a digitally augmented bicycle that aims to increase cyclists' motivation and social relatedness in physical activity. An experiment was conducted with a cycling simulation system. Both quantitative results and qualitative results show that SocialBike increased cyclists' intrinsic motivation, perceived competence, and social relatedness in physical activity.

References

1. Epstein, D.A., Jacobson, B.H., Bales, E., McDonald, D.W., Munson, S.A.: From nobody cares to way to go!: a design framework for social sharing in personal informatics. In: Proceedings of the 18th ACM Conference on Computer Supported Cooperative Work & Social Computing, pp. 1622–1636. ACM, February 2015
2. Pickett, C.L., Gardner, W.L., Knowles, M.: Getting a cue: the need to belong and enhanced sensitivity to social cues. Pers. Soc. Psychol. Bull. 30(9), 1095–1107 (2004)
3. Pickett, C.L., Gardner, W.L.: The Social Monitoring System: Enhanced Sensitivity to Social Cues as an Adaptive Response to Social Exclusion (2005)
4. Ivanov, A., Sharman, R., Rao, H.R.: Exploring factors impacting sharing health-tracking records. Health Policy Technol. 4(3), 263–276 (2015)
5. Curmi, F., Ferrario, M.A., Southern, J., Whittle, J.: HeartLink: open broadcast of live biometric data to social networks. In: Proceedings of the SIGCHI Conference on Human Factors in Computing Systems, pp. 1749–1758 (2013)
6. Mueller, F., Vetere, F., Gibbs, M.R., Edge, D., Agamanolis, S., Sheridan, J.G.: Jogging over a distance between Europe and Australia. In: Proceedings of the 23rd Annual ACM Symposium on User Interface Software and Technology, pp. 189–198. ACM, October 2010
7. Mauriello, M., Gubbels, M., Froehlich, J.E.: Social fabric fitness: the design and evaluation of wearable E-textile displays to support group running. In: Proceedings of the SIGCHI Conference on Human Factors in Computing Systems, pp. 2833–2842. ACM, April 2014
8. Walmink, W., Wilde, D., Mueller, F.F.: Displaying heart rate data on a bicycle helmet to support social exertion experiences. In: Proceedings of the 8th International Conference on Tangible, Embedded and Embodied Interaction, pp. 97–104. ACM, February 2014
9. Sonne, T., Jensen, M.M.: Race by hearts. In: Pisan, Y., Sgouros, N.M., Marsh, T. (eds.) ICEC 2014. LNCS, vol. 8770, pp. 125–132. Springer, Heidelberg (2014). https://doi.org/10.1007/978-3-662-45212-7_16
10. Beilharz, K.A., Moere, A.V., Stiel, B., Calò, C.A., Tomitsch, M., Lombard, A.: Expressive wearable sonification and visualisation: design and evaluation of a flexible display. In: NIME, pp. 323–326 (2010)

11. Walmink, W., Chatham, A., Mueller, F.: Interaction opportunities around helmet design. In: Extended Abstracts on Human Factors in Computing Systems, CHI 2014, pp. 367–370. ACM, April 2014
12. Liu, X., Vega, K., Qian, J., Paradiso, J., Maes, P.: Fluxa: body movements as a social display. In: Proceedings of the 29th Annual Symposium on User Interface Software and Technology, pp. 155–157. ACM, October 2016
13. Jacobs, M., Worbin, L.: Reach: dynamic textile patterns for communication and social expression. In: Extended Abstracts on Human Factors in Computing Systems, CHI 2005, pp. 1493–1496. ACM, April 2005
14. Kan, V., Fujii, K., Amores, J., Zhu Jin, C.L., Maes, P., Ishii, H.: Social textiles: social affordances and icebreaking interactions through wearable social messaging. In: Proceedings of the Ninth International Conference on Tangible, Embedded, and Embodied Interaction, pp. 619–624. ACM, January 2015
15. Genç, Ç., Erkaya, M., Balcı, F., Özcan, O.: Exploring dynamic expressions on soft wearables for physical exercises. In: Proceedings of the DIS 2018 Companion Publication of the 2018 Designing Interactive Systems Conference, pp. 147–152. ACM, May 2018
16. Laibowitz, M., Gips, J., Aylward, R., Pentland, A., Paradiso, J.A.: A sensor network for social dynamics. In: The Fifth International Conference on Information Processing in Sensor Networks, IPSN 2006, pp. 483–491. IEEE, April 2006
17. Yang, N., et al.: i-Ribbon: social expression through wearables to support weight-loss efforts. In: Intelligent Environments (Workshops), pp. 524–533 (2016)
18. Yang, N., van Hout, G., Feijs, L., Chen, W., Hu, J.: Eliciting values through wearable expression in weight loss. In: Proceedings of the 19th International Conference on Human-Computer Interaction with Mobile Devices and Services, p. 86. ACM, September 2017
19. Williams, A., Farnham, S., Counts, S.: Exploring wearable ambient displays for social awareness. In: Extended Abstracts on Human Factors in Computing Systems, CHI 2006, pp. 1529–1534. ACM, April 2006
20. Kleinman, L., Hirsch, T., Yurdana, M.: Exploring mobile devices as personal public displays. In: Proceedings of the 17th International Conference on Human-Computer Interaction with Mobile Devices and Services, pp. 233–243. ACM, August 2015
21. Pearson, J., Robinson, S., Jones, M.: It's about time: smartwatches as public displays. In: Proceedings of the 33rd Annual ACM Conference on Human Factors in Computing Systems, pp. 1257–1266. ACM, April 2015
22. Google Fit. https://developers.google.com/fit/
23. Yang, N., van Hout, G., Feijs, L., Chen, W., Hu, J.: Supporting weight loss through digitally-augmented social expression. In: Streitz, N., Konomi, S. (eds.) HCII 2019. LNCS, vol. 11587, pp. 459–470. Springer, Cham (2019). https://doi.org/10.1007/978-3-030-21935-2_35
24. Yang, N., van Hout, G., Feijs, L., Chen, W., Hu, J.: Simulating social cycling experience in design research. In: Ahram, T., Karwowski, W., Pickl, S., Taiar, R. (eds.) IHSED 2019. AISC, vol. 1026, pp. 379–384. Springer, Cham (2020). https://doi.org/10.1007/978-3-030-27928-8_58
25. McAuley, E., Duncan, T., Tammen, V.V.: Psychometric properties of the Intrinsic Motivation Inventory in a competitive sport setting: a confirmatory factor analysis. Res. Q. Exerc. Sport **60**(1), 48–58 (1989)

Assisting Radiologists in X-Ray Diagnostics

Cristian Avramescu⏺, Bercean Bogdan⏺, Stefan Iarca$^{(\boxtimes)}$⏺,
Andrei Tenescu⏺, and Sebastian Fuicu⏺

Politehnica University of Timisoara,
Piata Victoriei Nr. 2, 300006 Timisoara, Romania
stefan.iarca@student.upt.ro, sebastian.fuicu@cs.upt.ro

Abstract. Studies have shown that radiologists working together with Computer Aided Diagnostic software have increased accuracy. Automated screening software can be used to prioritize X-Rays coming in for diagnosis. We developed a suite of machine learning algorithms that aim to improve radiologist performance. It provides suggested diagnostics, a heatmap showing pathological areas and a bone subtracted version of the image which helps radiologists to identify fractures. We test different configurations for our diagnosis model, training it on both normal and enhanced images, using one or two branches. Our experiments show that adding enhanced inputs (lung segmented and bone subtracted versions of the input) increases the performance of our algorithm, which in turn increases the performance of the radiologist user. This shows that preprocessing the images before input increases model performance. More research is needed to find other preprocessing techniques, to refine existing ones, and to determine the optimal number and type of input X-Rays.

Keywords: Radiology · Deep Learning · X-ray · Segmentation · Bone · GAN

1 Introduction

In recent years, the decreasing costs and increasing efficiency of medical imaging equipment have made radiology a central tool in diagnosing diseases all around the world. X-rays are the most common form of medical imaging, with about 3.6 billion procedures performed yearly [1]. This large number can overcrowd radiologists, which decreases their diagnostic accuracy and can lead to fatigue [2].

We develop a suite of algorithms that aid radiologists in analyzing x-rays, by: screening the image and if any pathologies are found attempting to classify them into one of 13 classes, generating a heat-map of the diagnostic, lung segmenting the image, and creating a bone subtracted version of the image, which highlights the bone structure of the patient, making it easier to identify fractures.

N. M. Garcia et al. (Eds.): HealthyIoT 2019, LNICST 314, pp. 108–117, 2020.
https://doi.org/10.1007/978-3-030-42029-1_8

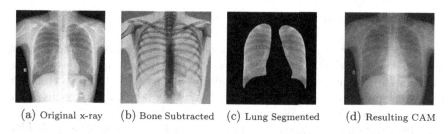

(a) Original x-ray   (b) Bone Subtracted   (c) Lung Segmented   (d) Resulting CAM

Fig. 1. Preprocessing steps and resulting class activation map

1.1 Related Work

CheXNet, described in [3], was not the first published approach to classifying diseases in X-rays. Many different network architectures have been developed for this task, such as CNN+RNN network, for exploiting the dependencies between labels [4], Cascading CNN with different loss functions [5], Attention Guided CNN [6].

The algorithms mentioned above use the ChestX-ray14 dataset, made available by [7], the first attempt of offering a large, labeled x-ray public dataset. Two new improved datasets have been published since: CheXpert [8] and MIMIC-CXR [9], totaling around 590.000 frontal and lateral chest x-rays.

Automatic lung segmentation has been studied for a long time. [10] used a gray level thresholding based approach. [11] proposed using a UNet combined with post processing methods to increase the segmentation accuracy. [12] explore different loss functions, and encoder pretraining.

Similarly, the field of bone supression has been explored for some time now. [13] attempt it using regression by k-nearest neighbor averaging, while [14] used multiple massive-trained artificial neural networks, a variant of fully connected networks. [15] suggests using Generative Adversarial Networks as a backbone for this task.

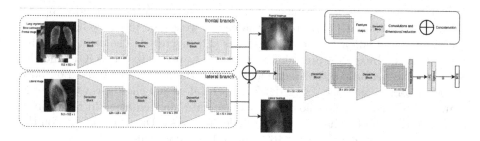

Fig. 2. Dual branch architecture

2 Our Contribution

In this work we create an end-to-end model for x-ray pathology classification based on the DenseNet-121 [16] architecture. We train it using custom augmentations on large public datasets, modify the network to support larger, 512×512 inputs and add bone subtracted and lung segmented versions of the inputs to increase accuracy. We propose a new dual branch architecture based on DenseNet-121 to increase accuracy in cases where lateral images are available.

The augmentation techniques we use to train all of our networks are based on [17]. We improve them by adding level adjustment, which is relevant for x-ray diagnostics and is used by radiologists in practice.

We add a stride 2 convolution and a stride 2 max pooling layer at the input of our DenseNet-121, to quickly reduce the dimensionality of our inputs from 512×512 to 128×128.

We trained 2 auxiliary models, a lung segmentation one (which increased our mean AUC by 0.004), and a bone subtraction one (which increases the average AUC by an additional 0.021). Coupled with our 2 branch architecture, this increases the mean AUC of our baseline by 0.038. Our current results are presented in Table 1.

3 Methods

3.1 Lung Segmentation

Lung segmentation is the task of extracting the lung area from an x-ray, removing areas that are considered irrelevant for diagnosing lung diseases. This can help radiologists better focus on the part of the image they are most interested in, as well as make it easier for them to take relevant measurements that they further use in the process of diagnostics.

Observing that lung segmentation would also reduce background noise for our pathology classification algorithm and help the model focus on more relevant areas, we set out to implement a model capable of segmentation (Fig. 1-c).

The model we train is built on a UNet [18] architecture. Instead of opting for the standard model described in the paper, we decide to use VGG16 [19] as the encoder and adapt the decoder to it, as [12] suggested. The main reason for this is that the ImageNet pretraining that can be applied to the VGG16 encoder improves the performance of the model. Unlike the author, we trained on both the Montgomery and the JSRT datasets, a total of 800 chest x-rays that were manually segmented by radiologists. We use data augmentation in the form of small rotations and translations. Our model achieves a Dice score of 0.96 on the validation dataset, consisting of 100 randomly sampled images.

One notable aspect of our training's results is that the model can achieve similar performance on datasets coming from different data distributions. Every x-ray generating machine generates radiographs slightly different, data coming from different machines varying in their distributions. Most of the CAD systems are not portable from one data distribution to another: the change makes them

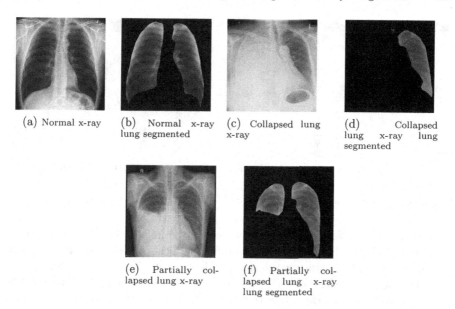

(a) Normal x-ray

(b) Normal x-ray lung segmented

(c) Collapsed lung x-ray

(d) Collapsed lung x-ray lung segmented

(e) Partially collapsed lung x-ray

(f) Partially collapsed lung x-ray lung segmented

Fig. 3. Limitations of the current lung segmentation algorithm

perform worse if the task they have to perform is non-trivial. The augmentation that we used, combined with the relative simplicity of the task and the use of 3 wildly different data distributions in the training dataset helped our model achieve a similar Dice score on other data.

A problem with this model, however, is that in case of lung obstruction, it will only partially segment the lungs. This can lead to downgraded performance down the line and is a good topic for further research. An example is shown in Fig. 3.

3.2 Bone Subtraction and Suppression

Bone subtracted x-rays are versions of the original images that strongly emphasize the skeletal tissue. They are useful in clinical settings as they help radiologists spot fractures and calcification signals, which can be hard to identify on the simple radiograph. They also present the advantage of being subtractive from the original radiograph, which leads to bone suppressed x-rays, in which the bone structure is not visible and the soft tissue can be seen better. Refer to Fig. 4.

The images are produced with the help of 'Dual Energy' enabled x-ray machines. Those expose the patient to two waves of radiation in an extremely fast sequence. The first wave has a higher dosage, while the second one is lower in intensity. This is the mechanism that allows the hardware to produce the bone subtracted image, and it is the most reliable way to obtain them (Fig. 1-b).

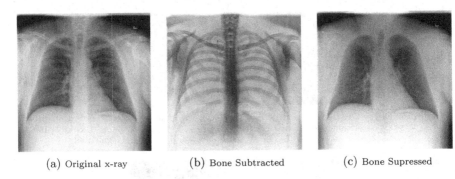

(a) Original x-ray   (b) Bone Subtracted   (c) Bone Supressed

Fig. 4. Bone subtraction and supression on an image from the ChestXRay-14 dataset

Our motivation for generating bone subtracted images with the help of artificial intelligence is that the method can yield an accuracy close to the one mentioned above while solving two major problems that standard hardware poses. The first one is that the second irradiation doesn't need to happen if using artificial intelligence, and the second is that 'Dual Energy' hardware is more expensive and not available as much as classic x-ray machines are.

To achieve the same effect as hardware techniques, we collect an anonymized dataset of 350 bone subtracted x-rays from the Oradea County Hospital. We use them to train a Conditional Deep Convolutional Generative Adversarial Network that can create a bone subtracted image. We start with the architecture of [15], and add [20]'s self attention, spectral normalization and update the discriminator and generator with the Two Times Update Rule (TTUR).

Doctors look after the contour of the bones when searching for fractures: thus, the resolution of the final image is extremely important. Our model benefits from adding a progressive multi-scaling strategy that helps it retain more of the exact structural information presented in the original radiograph.

After training our model and testing it on real cases, we conclude that the artificial intelligence, GAN technique can solve another problem that the hardware version encounters in practice: motion artifacts. The sequence of exposures of the 'Dual Energy' equipment is extremely fast, but the heart beating or slight movements of the patient can add artifacts to the image. While the full dataset that we have also contains artifact-broken images, we eliminate those and train on the 350 that contain little to no artifacts. The GAN model learns only from images without major artifacts and can generate artifact free bone subtracted images.

3.3   Pathology Classification

The most time consuming and important task of a radiologist with regards to x-ray analysis is diagnosing the study: identifying pathologies in the images at hand. Inspired by [3], we create an end-to-end classification model trained and validated on the official splits of the CheXPert and MIMIC-CXR datasets to help doctors with this difficult task.

We test multiple architectures like ResNet, Inception, VGG, and DenseNet. We conclude that DenseNet works best for our task and decide to use a DenseNet-121 architecture with 512×512 RGB image inputs as a baseline. The choice for a larger input image size slows down the training of the network, but the decision was driven by multiple consulations with radiologists. They suggested that smaller images do not retain enough detail on incipient pathologies or on ones that are well hidden.

Debugging neural networks is a notoriously difficult task, and artificial intelligence algorithms applied to clinical tasks have to be consistently stable and well tested before used in real scenarios. To see that the algorithm correctly links diagnostics to their appearances in the radiography, we explain its classification results by using the CAM [21] visualization technique. Some results are shown in Fig. 5.

We conclude that using this visualization method has two other benefits besides helping with debugging. It strengthens the doctor's trust in the CAD system, as he can see that the diagnostics the software suggests have good reasoning behind them, and it also guides doctors, after they gain trust in the model, to faster navigate the important areas of a radiographs.

We evaluate the model using the AUROC score (see Table 1), as it is the most widely used for quantifying results in this task.

Our baseline starts with ImageNet dataset pretraining. Because x-rays are very different from the images in the Imagenet [22] dataset, we decide to abandon the ImageNet transfer learning used by [3]. Instead, we develop a binary

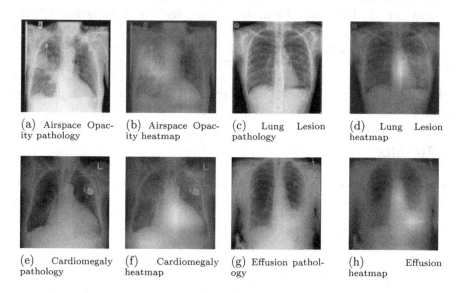

(a) Airspace Opacity pathology   (b) Airspace Opacity heatmap   (c) Lung Lesion pathology   (d) Lung Lesion heatmap

(e) Cardiomegaly pathology   (f) Cardiomegaly heatmap   (g) Effusion pathology   (h) Effusion heatmap

Fig. 5. Examples of pathologies and generated heatmaps

classification algorithm trained on the ChestX-ray14 dataset and use it to initialize the weights from our model. This greatly improves the speed at which the model reaches good performance and increases its AUROC score.

The binary classification model can tell normal radiographs apart from those that contain anomalies, without the ability to specify the exact anomaly that it encounters. While its main use was that of pretraining for our classification algorithm, we discuss possible use-cases with radiologists and reach the consensus that it is suitable for patient triage in highly dynamic and time-sensitive environments.

We train a binary classification algorithm and use it to initialize the weights of our model. The images resulting from our lung segmentation and GAN models provide valuable information to radiologists in real-world cases, so we decide to test if they help our model's performance as well.

To combine the images for the input, we switch to a single grayscale channel for the original x-ray image and add lung segmented and bone subtracted images (see Fig. 1) as inputs on separate channels.

Another tool used by radiologists in clinical scenarios is the lateral view radiographs. Some pathologies are not visible on frontal x-rays, while others can be hidden and can be seen more clearly with the help of a lateral investigation. With this in mind, we also add a second branch for a lateral chest x-ray, if one is available, believing that this will help the model associate anomalous areas in the frontal version with the ones present in the lateral version, for more accurate and comprehensive classification.

The lateral and frontal branches are constructed from 3 of the 5 Dense blocks normally used in DenseNet. Their outputs are firstly used to generate CAM visualization for both the images and are concatenated and fed into the last 2 Dense blocks, which provides enough depth for the network to learn correlations between the feature maps of the two branches.

Each of the images provides extra valuable information to the model, and adding them improves the model's performance. The architecture is described in Fig. 2.

4   Results

There are the results we obtained with different network and input configurations. There is a clear distinction in performance (as measured by the average AUC across all diseases) between them.

Table 1. AUC scores for various network architectures

Architecture	AUC score													
	AT	CA	CO	ED	PE	PN	PX	EC	LL	AO	PO	FR	SD	AVG
DN-121	0.827	0.813	0.827	0.892	0.922	0.716	0.812	0.795	0.675	0.752	0.822	0.494	0.849	0.784
DualBranch DN-121	0.843	0.831	0.837	0.910	0.934	0.733	0.817	0.814	0.683	0.763	0.828	0.500	0.866	0.797
+LungSegmentation	0.847	0.834	0.842	**0.913**	**0.938**	**0.735**	0.825	**0.817**	0.685	**0.773**	**0.833**	0.504	**0.871**	0.801
+BoneSubstracted	**0.851**	**0.841**	**0.845**	0.905	0.937	0.734	**0.827**	0.814	**0.693**	0.764	0.824	**0.784**	**0.871**	**0.822**

Classes: AT - Atelectasis; CA - Cardiomegaly; CO - Consolidation; ED - Edema; PE - Plerual Effusion; PN - Pneumonia; PX - Pneumothorax; EC - Enlarged Cardiomediastinum; LL - Lung Lesion; AO - Airspace Opacity; PO - Pleural Other; FR - Fracture; SD - Support Devices
DN-121 - baseline architecture, a DenseNet-121 with our initial downsampling layer, trained with augmented images
DualBranch DN-121 - our dual branch architecture, which takes 2 grayscale 1 channel inputs: frontal x-ray and lateral x-ray (if available)
+LungSegmentation - dual branch architecture, with an additional channel on the frontal input, which contains the lung segmented image
+BoneSubstracted - dual branch architecture + lung segmentation, with an additional channel on the frontal input, which contains bone subtracted images (see Fig. 2)

5 Discussion

Compared to other studies, by achieving a higher overall AUC we show that deep learning algorithms can benefit from learning with additional radiography information, which is natural because radiologists themselves find the auxiliary images useful.

Although we managed to increase our average AUC by combining different supplementary inputs, we were surprised to find that the AUC scores of some classes such as Edema and Pleural Effusion were decreased - this suggests that the dataset we are validating on has inconsistencies in how accurate the classes it contains are obtained.

This uncovers a major limitation of this study: the dataset used for training is labeled with NLP algorithms which provide an effective way of creating a large database of images and labels, but not an error-prone one. We believe a sharp rise in the algorithm performance could be provided by a radiologist hand-labeled dataset and we think that using such a dataset at least for validation is a necessity in future works.

6 Conclusion

In conclusion, we manage to improve the performance of our baseline model by increasing the size of the input, tweaking the DenseNet backbone, using weight initialization from a task performed on the same data distribution and by adding as inputs supplementary images, created by our 2 auxiliary models, that hold valuable information about the case. The lung segmentation model performs well on different data distributions than the ones it was trained on, while the GAN model that generates bone subtracted images from classic x-rays can solve a problem that consecrated hardware methods encounter: motion-artifacts.

In the future we plan to investigate what other auxiliary images can help the model learn even more detail about the x-ray it has to interpret, as well as to improve the backbone architecture by adding attention modules and investigating multi-task learning approaches.

Lung Masks for Shenzhen Hospital Chest X-ray (Montgomery) Set:

– Dataset: https://www.kaggle.com/eduardomineo/u-net-lung-segmentation-montgomery-shenzhen/data
– Data Sources
  • National Library of Medicine, National Institutes of Health, Bethesda, MD, USA;
  • Computer Engineering Department, Faculty of Informatics and Computer Engineering, National Technical University of Ukraine "Igor Sikorsky Kyiv Polytechnic Institute", Kyiv, Ukraine;
– Works using this dataset:
  • Jaeger S, Karargyris A, Candemir S, Folio L, Siegelman J, Callaghan F, Xue Z, Palaniappan K, Singh RK, Antani S, Thoma G, Wang YX, Lu PX, McDonald CJ. Automatic tuberculosis screening using chest radiographs. IEEE Trans Med Imaging 2014;33:233-45.
  • Candemir S, Jaeger S, Palaniappan K, Musco JP, Singh RK, Xue Z, Karargyris A, Antani S, Thoma G, McDonald CJ. Lung segmentation in chest radiographs using anatomical atlases with nonrigid registration. IEEE Trans Med Imaging 2014;33:577-90.
  • Yu. Gordienko, Yu. Kochura, O. Alienin, O. Rokovyi, S. Stirenko, Peng Gang, Wei Zeng, Chest X-Ray Analysis of Tuberculosis by Deep Learning with Segmentation and Augmentation, arXiv preprint arXiv:1803.01199 (2018).

JSRT dataset: Japanese Society of Radiological Technology

– https://www.jsrt.or.jp/data/english/jsrt/.

References

1. PAHO WHO. World Radiography Day: Two-Thirds of the World's Population has no Access to Diagnostic Imaging. PAHO (2012)
2. Stec, N., Arje, D., Moody, A.R., Krupinski, E.A., Tyrrell, P.N.: A systematic review of fatigue in radiology: is it a problem? AJR Am. J. Roentgenol. **210**(4), 799–806 (2018)
3. Rajpurkar, P., et al.: CheXNet: Radiologist-Level Pneumonia Detection on Chest X-Rays with Deep Learning. arXiv e-prints, art. arXiv:1711.05225, November 2017
4. Yao, L., Poblenz, E., Dagunts, D., Covington, B., Bernard, D., Lyman, K.: Learning to diagnose from scratch by exploiting dependencies among labels. arXiv e-prints, art. arXiv:1710.10501, October 2017
5. Kumar, P., Grewal, M., Srivastava, M.M.: Boosted Cascaded Convnets for Multilabel Classification of Thoracic Diseases in Chest Radiographs. arXiv e-prints, art. arXiv:1711.08760, November 2017
6. Guan, Q., Huang, Y., Zhong, Z., Zheng, Z., Zheng, L., Yang, Y.: Diagnose like a Radiologist: Attention Guided Convolutional Neural Network for Thorax Disease Classification. arXiv e-prints, art. arXiv:1801.09927, January 2018

7. Wang, X., Peng, Y., Lu, L., Lu, Z., Bagheri, M., Summers, R.M.: ChestX-ray8: Hospital-scale Chest X-ray Database and Benchmarks on Weakly-Supervised Classification and Localization of Common Thorax Diseases. arXiv e-prints, art. arXiv:1705.02315, May 2017

8. Irvin, J., et al.: CheXpert: A Large Chest Radiograph Dataset with Uncertainty Labels and Expert Comparison. arXiv e-prints, art. arXiv:1901.07031, January 2019

9. Johnson, A.E.W., et al.: MIMIC-CXR: a large publicly available database of labeled chest radiographs. arXiv e-prints, art. arXiv:1901.07042, January 2019

10. Armato III, S.G., Giger, M.L., MacMahon, H.: Automated lung segmentation in digitized posteroanterior chest radiographs. Acad. Radiol. **5**(4), 245–255 (1998)

11. Rashid, R., Akram, M.U., Hassan, T.: Fully convolutional neural network for lungs segmentation from chest X-rays. In: Campilho, A., Karray, F., ter Haar Romeny, B. (eds.) ICIAR 2018. LNCS, vol. 10882, pp. 71–80. Springer, Cham (2018). https://doi.org/10.1007/978-3-319-93000-8_9. ISBN 978-3-319-93000-8

12. Frid-Adar, M., Ben-Cohen, A., Amer, R., Greenspan, H.: Improving the Segmentation of Anatomical Structures in Chest Radiographs using U-Net with an ImageNet Pre-trained Encoder. arXiv e-prints, art. arXiv:1810.02113, October 2018

13. Loog, M., van Ginneken, B., Schilham, A.M.R.: Filter learning: application to suppression of bony structures from chest radiographs. Med. Image Anal. **10**(6), 826–840 (2006). https://doi.org/10.1016/j.media.2006.06.002. http://www.sciencedirect.com/science/article/pii/S1361841506000454. ISSN 1361-8415

14. Chen, S., Suzuki, K.: Separation of bones from chest radiographs by means of anatomically specific multiple massive-training anns combined with total variation minimization smoothing. IEEE Trans. Med. Imaging **33**(2), 246–257 (2014). https://doi.org/10.1109/TMI.2013.2284016

15. Zhou, B., Lin, X., Eck, B., Hou, J., Wilson, D.: Generation of virtual dual energy images from standard single-shot radiographs using multi-scale and conditional adversarial network. In: Jawahar, C.V., Li, H., Mori, G., Schindler, K. (eds.) ACCV 2018. LNCS, vol. 11361, pp. 298–313. Springer, Cham (2019). https://doi.org/10.1007/978-3-030-20887-5_19

16. Huang, G., Liu, Z., van der Maaten, L., Weinberger, K.Q.: Densely Connected Convolutional Networks. arXiv e-prints, art. arXiv:1608.06993, August 2016

17. He, T., Zhang, Z., Zhang, H., Zhang, Z., Xie, J., Li, M.: Bag of Tricks for Image Classification with Convolutional Neural Networks. arXiv e-prints, art. arXiv:1812.01187, December 2018

18. Ronneberger, O., Fischer, P., Brox, T.: U-Net: Convolutional Networks for Biomedical Image Segmentation. arXiv e-prints, art. arXiv:1505.04597, May 2015

19. Simonyan, K., Zisserman, A.: Very Deep Convolutional Networks for Large-Scale Image Recognition. arXiv e-prints, art. arXiv:1409.1556, September 2014

20. Zhang, H., Goodfellow, I., Metaxas, D., Odena, A.: Self-Attention Generative Adversarial Networks. arXiv e-prints, art. arXiv:1805.08318, May 2018

21. Zhou, B., Khosla, A., Lapedriza, A., Oliva, A., Torralba, A.: Learning Deep Features for Discriminative Localization. arXiv e-prints, art. arXiv:1512.04150, December 2015

22. Deng, J., Dong, W., Socher, R., Li, L.-J., Li, K., Fei-Fei, L.: ImageNet: a large-scale hierarchical image database. In: CVPR 2009 (2009)

Design and Evaluation for Digital Forensic Ready Wireless Medical Systems

Ar Kar Kyaw, Zhuang Tian$^{(\boxtimes)}$, and Brian Cusack

Digital Forensic Research Laboratory, School of Engineering,
Computer and Mathematical Science, Auckland University of Technology,
55 Wellesley Street East, Auckland, New Zealand
{arkar.kyaw,zhuang.tian,brian.cusack}@aut.ac.nz

Abstract. This paper reports research into mitigating security vulnerability in IoT medical devices by inserting forensic readiness states into the network system and preparing mitigation for security failure. A design is built and tested, and then validated by expert feedback. The contribution of this research is to present a novel conceptual design for a digital forensic readiness framework for WMedSys, which can be easily implemented and integrated into existing IoT and wireless networks in the healthcare sector.

Keywords: IoT · Wireless · Medical · Forensic · Readiness · Framework

1 Introduction

Internet of things (IoT) have become a critical part of the way people live and work. In the last of few years, IoT devices have started playing more important roles, and even providing vital services to companies, enterprises, government departments, healthcare and public sectors [1]. However, security incidents are rapidly increasing along with the benefits provided by IoT. In expectations of information system (IS) security incident response (Request for Comments: RFC 2350), Brownlee and Guttman [2] define security incidents as "any adverse event which compromises some aspect of computer or network security" (p. 17). Hence, a security or cyber security incident is commonly associated with the compromise of the pillars of network security such as confidentiality, integrity, availability, authentication, and the like. For example, the manipulation or alteration of patient data from the personal health record (PHR) or electronic medical record (EMR) of a hospital or a clinical network in the healthcare sector is one of the compromises of network security. Currently, the approach deployed, or action taken by organisations or government departments to mitigate cyber security incidents is oriented to disaster recovery and business continuity to lessen the impact on business processes [3]. But, the impact on business processes can also be reduced by having a digital forensic readiness (DFR) system. Having a DFR system in an organisation is "having an appropriate level of capability in order to be able to preserve, collect, protect and analyse digital evidence so that this evidence can be used effectively: in any legal matters; in security investigations; in disciplinary proceeding; in an employment tribunal; or in a court of law" [4, p. 3]. In fact, the DFR system can help an organisation not only to properly acquire and preserve digital evidence (DE), but also to simplify the digital forensic investigation (DFI) process after a security incident happens. In addition, the DFR system can help an organisation to reduce cost, optimise the time and have digital evidence that could be acceptable by a court of law.

Over the last decade, the number of cyber incidents in the healthcare environment including hospitals that deployed wireless medical networks (WMedSys) and wireless medical devices (WMedDs) have significantly increased due to malicious internal and external attacks. For instance, Quinn [5] reported that Hancock Health Regional Hospital from Greenfield (Indiana, United States) paid a small ransom ($55,000.00) to the hackers to regain access to its computer systems due to over 1,400 files being encrypted by ransomware. Similarly, one recent cyber incident was when an authorised employee stole 28,434 patients' related data and their sensitive records from the Centre for Health Care Services in San Antonio in December 2017 [6]. Such incidents are occurring and becoming part of any organisation or healthcare environment that claim to invest in the best technology and resources to provide unfeasible 100 percent security for its information system. In fact, there are many security threats and risks (such as human errors, DDoS and MITM attacks) to the WMedSys and WMedDs [7–12]. Therefore, it is essential to have a proper DFR system for investigating security incidents [13]. As a result, different researchers have proposed theoretical frameworks for forensic readiness of cloud computing [14–18], a theoretical forensic model for acquiring digital evidence in the Internet of Things (IoT) [19] and a theoretical network forensic readiness framework for generic enterprise networks [20]. Moreover, some researchers [21] introduce a generic DFR model for Bring-Your-Own-Device (BYOD) to capture potential (DE by utilising Honeypot while others propose a mobile DFR model [22] and a DFR framework for small to medium-sized enterprise (SME) environments [23]. Similarly, Ngobeni, Venter, and Burke [24] present a prototype implementation of a forensic readiness model for WLANs whereas Rahman, Ahmad and Ramli [25] designed a DFR for WBAN based on the previous proposed research [26]. However, to the best of our knowledge, none of the previous research focuses on the DFR of a hospital wireless network (WMedSys) that deploys WPA2-Enterprise for handling security attacks (such as MITM, patient data manipulation, etc.). Consequently, we extend our proposed DFR of WMedSys [26] to address the research gap. Therefore, the main contribution in this paper is to design and evaluate a novel DFR framework for WMedSys. Hence, the structure of this paper is as follows. Section 2 provides the background of DF, DFR and the significance of DFR. Sections 3 and 4 present the research methodology and the conceptual design of the proposed DFR framework for WMedSys, respectively. Section 5 explains the conceptual design of the proposed DFR framework artefact, which is followed by findings and discussion in Sect. 6. Finally, we discuss limitations and future work in the conclusion (Sect. 7).

2 Background

Any information system including WMedSys is susceptible to cyber-attacks or incidents due vulnerabilities such as technical flaws and weakness of users who use those systems. For example, different researchers have demonstrated attacks in wireless networks as a result of the technical flaws in wireless security protocols (WEP, WPA or WPA2). Thus, any malicious person or adversary can exploit these vulnerabilities in order to destroy, manipulate or steal confidential data of an organisation. In such situations, the impact of cyber-attacks can lead the organisation to have financial and reputation losses. In a severe case scenario, the life of a patient or a person who uses a WMedD (e.g. continuous wireless glucose monitoring system or wireless implantable medical device) could be in serious danger if the patient's physiological data from WMedSys or WMedD is compromised. As a consequence, the DF investigator has to investigate the cyber incident by applying DFI processes in order to answer questions related to the case under investigation. Ieong [27, p. S33] describes six categories of questions in the "FORZA (FORensics Zachman framework)" paper, including "Why (the motivation), What (the data), How (the procedures), Where (the location), Who (the people), and When (the time)" that are related to the eight DF investigator roles. However, the time taken (cost) to perform the investigation and the possibility of failure to collect DE related to the cyber indent or crime could be high if a proper DFR system is not in place. Therefore, this section provides a brief introduction to digital forensics, digital forensic readiness (DFR) and its significance, the requirements of DFR, and attacks in WMedSys and WMedDs.

2.1 Digital Forensics

DF is an emerging area and has many definitions. DF is defined as "the use of scientifically derived and proven methods toward the preservation, collection, validation, identification, analysis, interpretation, documentation and presentation of digital evidence derived from digital sources for the purpose of facilitation or furthering the reconstruction of events found to be criminal, or helping to anticipate unauthorized actions shown to be disruptive to planned operations." In NIST Special Publication (800-86: Guide to Integrating Forensic Techniques into Incident Response), Kent et al. [29, p. E-11] defines DF as computer and network forensics that apply "science to the identification, collection, examination, and analysis of data while preserving the integrity of the information and maintaining a strict chain of custody for the data or digital information". Similarly, other researchers describe DF as "a branch of forensic science focusing on the recovery and investigation of raw data residing in electronic or digital devices (p. 8)". Nonetheless, DF necessitates a high level of attentiveness and accuracy to ensure the evidential data is uncompromised, reliable and verifiable during the course of investigation. As a result, it is essential to have a DFR system in WMedSys for preserving the integrity potential digital evidence that can be admissible in a court of law. The following sub-sections explain DFR and the significance of having a DFR system in organisations.

2.2 Digital Forensic Readiness

Unlike digital forensic investigations (DFI), DFR is a proactive measure that healthcare providers such as clinics or hospitals have to enforce and implement in order "to comply to DFI with sufficient forensic preparedness" [18, p. 25]. The main objective of DFR is to achieve maximum capability of any healthcare provider in collecting potential digital evidence related to cyber incidents or digital crimes while reducing the cost of DFI during investigations [14, 16, 23, 31–33]. Similarly, ISO/IEC 27043 highlights DFR as a process that focuses on pre-incident investigation [2014, cited in 21]. DFR can be defined as "the achievement of an appropriate level of capability by an organisation in order for it to be able to collect, preserve, protect and analyse digital evidence so that this evidence can be effectively used in any legal matters, disciplinary matters, employment tribunal or court of law" [CESG, Good Practice Guide No. 18, cited in 3, p. 1; 35, p. 1]. Some researchers [18, 21, 22] state that DFR is the dynamic process in which an organisation requires forensic planning and preparation for collecting, accumulating and processing incident response data. In fact, a forensic readiness plan can help organisations not only to fulfil a compliance requirement, but also to provide potential evidence during DFI as part of internal investigation [35]. Other researchers [36] describe DFR as one of the metrics that organisations can use to measure its ability to thwart cybercrimes. Moreover, DFR's goal is to maximise the utilisation of preserved digital evidence if any information security incident happens within the organisation [16, 37]. In addition, Carrier and Spafford [2003, cited in 9] define DFR as "pre-incident plan within the digital forensic (DF) lifecycle that deals with DF identification, preservation, and storage whilst minimising the costs of a forensic investigation (p. 1)". The pre-incident plan of pro-active DF can also empower an organisation to be DFR and provide DFR as an integral component of an information system's best practice [32]. Hence, DFR of a WMedSys can be defined as a mechanism or system that can provide the capability to collect potential digital evidence related to cyber incidents or digital crimes while reducing the cost of DF during investigations.

2.3 Significance of Digital Forensic Readiness

The significance of having a DFR system in organisations has been stated by many researchers. A DFR system can be usually implemented as a pre-incident mechanism to collect and preserve potential DE while reducing the DF investigation cost by promptly and effectively responding to a cyber incident [24, 39–41]. Regiani [3] mentions that a DFR system can help organisations to simplify activities and reduce the process or step for collecting the DE during DFI. In applying a DFR framework, the authors [38] discuss that a DFR can complement the information security policy of an organisation by proactively practising its forensic capability in DE collection. In addition, any organisation with a DFR system deployed will be complying with legal preparedness when it comes to dealing with cybercrime or digital crime cases [18, 20, 33], as the organisation can rapidly collect, inspect, analyse and report the credible DE related to the cybercrime case under investigation. Due to the advances in technology, Pooe and Labuschagne [42] and Rowlingson [33] also state that there is a need to review and enhance DF models and processes, which can support organisations in finding DE quickly and allow the validation of DE easily. Similarly, other researchers [23] point out that having a DFR system can benefit organisations in collecting DE without disruption or minimising the effect to the operation of organisations during investigation and ensure the collected DE has an impact on the outcome of any legal progress. Therefore, the organisation will be well prepared to get the reliable DE at a lower cost [14, 31, 33, 40] and will have the best response [37, 43] when a cyber incident happens. In fact, the DFR system must be capable of logging or preserving the digital footprints linking to users' activities including authorised (internal) or unauthorised (external) malicious actions within the organisation's IT environment. The digital footprints should disclose details of the malicious person or user account, the source (such as originated IP and MAC addresses), the type or technique used, and date and time of an attack [9, 44]. Moreover, Rowlingson [33] introduced "a ten-step process for forensic readiness", in which the importance of having a DFR system is evidently stated. Therefore, DE is admissible in a court of law, organisations can appreciate the significance of the "legal sensitivities of evidence [33, p. 1]", and the organisation can maximise "ability to collect credible digital evidence and minimise the cost of an internal investigation during an incident response (p. 3)". Likewise, Rowlingson highlights the DFR can help organisations in utilising it "as a deterrent to insider threat", demonstrating "due diligence and good corporate governance of the company's information assets", signifying "regulatory requirements have been met", improving "the prospects for a successful legal action", or resolving "a commercial dispute", and lessening "interruption to the business from any investigation" (pp. 6–9). Previous researchers [17] also raised the importance of having proactive DFR system in the cloud computing environment for gathering potential evidence or valuable data pertaining to cyber incidents for saving time and money during DFI. However, other researchers [20] raise the point that the DFR is a resource intensive answer to DFI even though the DFR can reduce the incident response cost and provide "the basis for security awareness training throughout the enterprise (p. 6)". Nonetheless, the DFR can safeguard against security attacks or breaches by adding appropriate security controls, ensure good corporate information security (IS) governance is in practice to effectively verify possible sources of any security attacks, and provide the IS strategy enhancement of an organisation [32, 34]. Furthermore, having a DFR system in any organisation or in the WMedSys of a healthcare provider can fulfil not only the requirements of DE preservation [33, 34, 45], but also the prevention of a cyber incident from happening within an organisation [15, 34].

3   Research Methodology

3.1   Design Science Research Paradigm

The design science (DS) is a paradigm "for developing scientific knowledge about the problem domain, including artefact, and engineering knowledge about carrying out design" [46, p. 134]. However, Fleming [46] claims that the DS paradigm provides the way in which the process of research should progress and what is required to be addressed in the research to assure its quality instead of giving the direction on how the artefact should be designed. Moreover, Fleming [46] also argues that the research rigour requirements are commonly in conflict with a major requirement of DS, which is related to real business problems. As a result, a DS paradigm should provide a framework that addresses the problems related to research rigour rather than specifying rigour requirements.

3.2   Design Science Research Methodology

Design science research methodology (DSRM) is proposed by Peffers et al. [47, p. 1] in order to achieve "a commonly accepted framework for DSR" by integrating "principles, practices, and procedures required to carry out DSR" in information systems. To provide a proof of concept, the proposed DSRM is evaluated by using four IS case studies. There are six process elements in the proposed DSRM (see Fig. 1) which are based on well- accepted elements and are derived from previously published papers.

The first process of the DSRM is the "problem identification and motivation" as it is important to define the particular research problem that will be employed in the development of an artefact, which can present a solution effectively. However, the value of such a solution can be achieved by motivating "the researcher and the audience of the research to pursue the solution and to accept the results and it helps to understand the reasoning associated with the researcher's understanding of the problem [47, p. 55]". Hence, the knowledge of the state of the problem and the importance of its solution are required resources in this process stage.

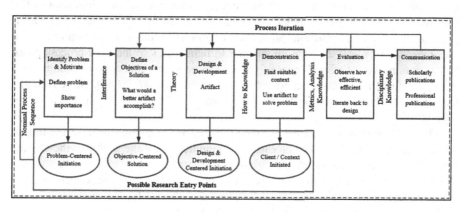

Fig. 1. Design science research methodology process model [47, p. 54]

The second process of DSRM is to "define the objectives for a solution" from the definition of the problem and knowledge of feasibility. The objectives should be deduced from the problem specification and could be quantitative or qualitative. For instance, the quantitative objective can be "a desirable solution would be better than current ones [47, p. 55]". Similar to the first process stage, the knowledge of the state of problems and current solutions, if any, and their efficacy are required as resources in this process stage.

The third process is to "design and develop" the artefact, which can be "constructs, models, methods, or instantiations" or "new properties of technical, social or informational resources [Jarvinen, 2007, p. 49 cited 48, p. 55]. According to Peffers et al. [47] a conceptual DS artefact is an artefact in which a research contribution is embedded in the design. The architecture and desired or required functionality of the artefact is indispensable for creating the tangible artefact, and therefore theory knowledge is an essential resource that can bring in a solution.

The fourth process is the "demonstration" of the artefact application in order to answer one or more cases of the problem by using "experimentation, simulation, case study, proof or other appropriate method [47, p. 55]". Thus, the effective knowledge for utilising the artefact to answer the problem is an important resource in this process stage.

The fifth process is the "evaluation", in which how well the artefact provides a solution to the problem (effectiveness and efficiency) can be observed and measured by evaluating "the objectives of a solution to actual observed results from the use of artefact in the demonstration" [47, p. 56]. As a result, the knowledge of relevant metrics and analysis methods are necessary in this stage. However, the artefact evaluation may be different depending upon the nature of the problem context. For instance, the evaluation may be done by comparing the functionality of the artefact with the solution objectives from the second process of the DSRM process model in addition to other quantitative evaluation methods such as surveys, client feedback, or simulations [47]. Nevertheless, the evaluation should conceptually consist of any suitable empirical or pragmatic evidence or plausible proof. After completing the evaluation process, the researchers can make a decision on whether to iterate back to the third process phase "to try to improve the effectiveness of the artefact or to continue on to communication and leave further improvement to subsequent projects" [47, p. 56]. Moreover, the feasibility of iteration will be based on the nature of the research in the problem context.

The final process of the DSRM process model is "communication" according to previous researchers. Thus, the problem, the significance of the problem, the artefact designed, the utility and novelty, the rigor of the artefact design and its effectiveness should be communicated "to researchers and other relevant audiences such as practicing professionals, when appropriate" [47, p. 56]. Similarly, the outcome of DSR could be communicated in scholarly research publications (Fig. 2).

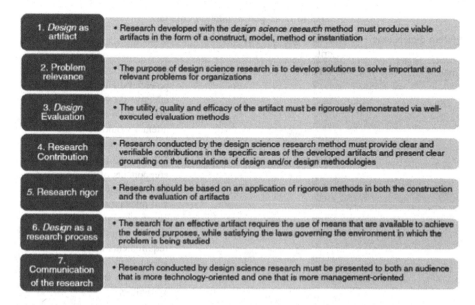

1. *Design* as artifact	• Research developed with the *design science research* method must produce viable artifacts in the form of a construct, model, method or instantiation
2. Problem relevance	• The purpose of design science research is to develop solutions to solve important and relevant problems for organizations
3. *Design* Evaluation	• The utility, quality and efficacy of the artifact must be rigorously demonstrated via well-executed evaluation methods
4. Research Contribution	• Research conducted by the design science research method must provide clear and verifiable contributions in the specific areas of the developed artifacts and present clear grounding on the foundations of design and/or design methodologies
5. Research rigor	• Research should be based on an application of rigorous methods in both the construction and the evaluation of artifacts
6. *Design* as a research process	• The search for an effective artifact requires the use of means that are available to achieve the desired purposes, while satisfying the laws governing the environment in which the problem is being studied
7. Communication of the research	• Research conducted by design science research must be presented to both an audience that is more technology-oriented and one that is more management-oriented

Fig. 2. Design science research methodology process model [47, p. 54]

3.3 Artefact Evaluation Criteria

According to March and Smith (1995), the main purpose of evaluation in Design Science Research (DSR) is to ensure the goal that an artefact design aligns with the solution of an identified problem and controls the progress of design development and deployment of an artefact. To systematically review whether the progress has been accomplished or completed, evaluation criteria should be formulated. Hence, March and Smith suggest a set of evaluation criteria for DSR artefacts.

Nonetheless, researchers not only need to focus on academic interest, but also more importantly need to consider the industry application and adoption of an artefact. Such an implication is the essential goal of DSR. For example, on the one hand, industry is more concerned with how easy an artefact can be used, how well it can be adopted and how efficient it can be. On the other hand, researcher is more interested in how reliable the artefact is and whether or not it is adequate. Therefore, when selecting the evaluation criteria and subsequently formulating evaluation questions, a researcher must satisfy both needs and only ask relevant and appropriated questions to ensure the process will be conducted thoroughly and rigorously.

In addition, another set of evaluation criteria has been developed by Rosemann and Vessey [9]. These criteria focus on whether or not an artefact can be applicable to an industry practitioner. These criteria include importance, suitability and accessibility of an artefact. Further, Prat et al. (2014) have recommended a new set of criteria based on March and Smith [1] for evaluating information systems (IS) artefacts which is comprised of three major components including system dimensions, evaluation criteria and sub-criteria. The new set of evaluation criteria introduces more categories and further divides March & Smith's criteria into a hierarchical set. Thus, it provides more precise and balanced evaluation result against an artefact. Table 1 shows artefact evaluation criteria based on a systematic approach derived from Prat et al. (2014).

Table 1. Expert evaluation criteria

System dimensions	Evaluation criteria	Sub-criteria	Questions
Goal	Efficacy		Q1: Overall, for preserving potential digital evidence, how effective do you think the proposed DFR Framework artefact would be in the production environment?
	Validity		Q2: Are the defined components of the proposed DFR Framework artefact clear and relevant to what you observe? Q3: Do you think the provided requirements helpful and adequate in designing DFR Framework artefact for WMedSys?
Environment	Consistency with people	Utility	Q9: Do you think the proposed DFR Framework is effective and efficient in capturing security attacks on a WMedSys? Q10: Do you think the proposed DFR Framework is effective and efficient in determining security attacks on a WMedSys? Q11: Do you think the proposed DFR Framework is effective and efficient in addressing to improve patient/user safety? Q18: How effective do you think the proposed DFR Framework could be if IT managers/security engineers of clinical and hospital networks start using it in their WMedSys?
		Understandability	Q6. What was an approximate time for you to follow all components of proposed DFR Framework artefact? Was it easy to understand?

(continued)

Table 1. (*continued*)

System dimensions	Evaluation criteria	Sub-criteria	Questions
			Q15. Were the information provided related to the artefact logical and helpful?
		Ease of use	Q5: How easy or difficult do you think it is to implement and integrate the proposed DFR Framework artefact in an existing WMedSys? Q12: Please provide your comments on the usability and ease of operation
	Consistency with organization	Utility	Q4: Do you think the proposed artefact is useful and realistic in improving/addressing user/patient safety? Q16: Is the proposed DFR Framework artefact cost effective and efficient? Q17: Is the proposed artefact likely to be widely adopted and implemented in WMedSys?
Structure & Activity (Dynamic, the operations and functionalities of the artefact)	Completeness		Q7: Do you think there is any area of improvement in the proposed artefact? If so, please give your suggestion Q8: Is there any modification that should be made to any component of the proposed DFR Framework? Q13: Can you list the weaknesses and strengths of the proposed DFR Framework artefact for WMedSys? Q14: Regarding the completeness of the DFR Framework artefact for WMedSys, how do you think?

4 Conceptual Design of the Proposed Framework Artefact

The proposed DFR Framework artefact for WMedSys (see Fig. 3) is composed of several components such as Pi-drone, Wireless Forensic Server (WFS), Remote Authentication Dial-In User Service (RADIUS) Server, Wireless Access Point (WAP) Controller,

Integrity Checking/Hashing Server (OSSEC), Intrusion Detection/Prevention System (Bro-IDS) Server, Web Server (XAMPP), and a centralised Syslog Server (Splunk).

Pi-drone: It uses the Kali Linux ARM version to act as a forensic wireless drone. Kali Linux is Debian-based Linux distribution which contains many tools designed for penetrating testing and security audits. A TP-link Wi-Fi USB was connected to the Raspberry Pi to use to scan the Wi-Fi signal on 2.4 GHz. Pi-drone also utilises Kismet application which can sense any wireless network device detector, sniffer, wardriving tool, and WIDS (wireless intrusion detection) framework. By using Kismet as drone mode, Pi-drone can scan and capture the wireless signal coming from any Wi-Fi devices then all the information collected will be sent to a Wireless Forensic Server for analysis.

Wireless Forensic Server (WFS): It uses the Kali Linux operating system and runs Kismet application as a wireless intrusion detection system (WIDS) server. The Kismet server receives, categorises and analyses the information sent by Pi-drones. The server lists the wireless access points (APs) based on the service set identifiers (SSIDs) and their associated Media Access Control (MAC) addresses. Moreover, it also presents all clients including clients' MAC addresses connected to the same SSID (Kismetwireless, 2019). WFS server hosted a database which stores all the legitimate APs and clients' MAC addresses. The server will then forward all the logs with different information (e.g. timestamps, clients' MAC address, brute force attack timestamps). WFS can identify different brute force attacks on the wireless client as soon as it detects the attacks. In addition, the source code of Kismet can be modified to add new capabilities to detect different wireless attacks. Then, all the information will be forwarded to the Syslog server for further investigation.

Remote Authentication Dial-In User Service (RADIUS) Server: The main purpose of a RADIUS server is to provide the authentication service for user's network connection requests and return appropriate configuration information, accordingly. By using a Microsoft Windows Server 2008R2 for RADIUS server, RADIUS controls devices and user's authentication based on the username and password stored on the Domain Controller server. In this proposed DFR Framework, all the information and log (including username, timestamp, client MAC address) of the RADIUS server will be forwarded to the Syslog server as soon as a wireless client is successfully or unsuccessfully connected to the legitimate AP.

Access Point Controller (Unifi controller): A Microsoft Windows Server 2008R2 hosts the UniFi Controller software. This software controls and monitors all the Unifi APs on the network, decides the SSID on each APs based on different VLAN. It also monitors clients connected to each APs and SSIDs. In this proposed DFR Framework, the server will forward all the logs (e.g. AP MAC address a client connected to, timestamp, and client MAC address) to the Syslog server.

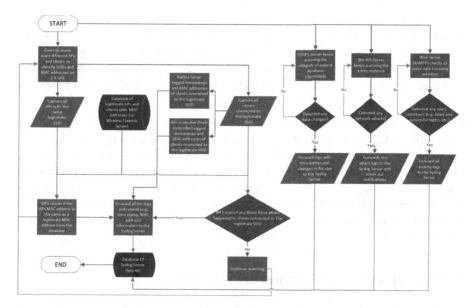

Fig. 3. Digital forensic readiness framework for WMedSys

Integrity Checking/Hashing Server (OSSEC) Server: OSSEC is a widely used scalable open-source application for the Host-based Intrusion Detection System (HIDS), which can run on different operating system platforms. It provides extensive features such as file integrity checking, Windows registry monitoring, rootkit detection, real-time alerting and active response. The security requirements can be tailored through configuration options and customised rules can be added. For example, OSSEC scripts can be written to perform actions responding to security alerts. In addition, the source code of OSSEC can be modified to add new capabilities. In this proposed DFR Framework, OSSEC is used to check the integrity of the patient's database (need to specify where that database is located, e.g. OpenEMR runs on which machine). Any change in patient-related data will be logged. Those logs comprise of timestamps, hash values, and changes in file sizes. Then, all information is configured to be forwarded to the Syslog server.

IDS Server (Bro-IDS): The IDS server runs Bro-IDS on top of Ubuntu OS. Bro-IDS is a passive, open-source network traffic analyser. Its primary function is to provide security monitoring and inspection of all traffic for signs of suspicious activity. Furthermore, it supports various traffic analysis tasks including performance measurements and helping with trouble-shooting (Zeek, 2019). In this proposed DFR Framework, Bro-IDS continues scanning the entire network to identify any attacks on the network such as a Distributed Denial-of-Service (DDoS) attack, and network scanning. All the information collected by the server will be forwarded to the Syslog server.

Web Server (XAMPP): It is a compilation of free software (comparable to a Linux distribution) (Apachefriends, 2019). XAMPP provides a web server platform which allows the hosting of any website or web service in low cost. This server hosts OpenEMR which provides patient related electronic medical records (OpenEMR, 2018) and provides a platform for users to use a different function from OpenEMR. In this proposed DFR Framework, all the users' activities (e.g. user success and failure logins, setting changes, and timestamp) will be logged by XAMPP and then forwarded to the Syslog server.

Syslog Server (Splunk): Splunk is a commercial software which is designed to collect and analysed data from different devices, and software on the network system. The Splunk server will be run on a Windows Server 2008R2 and in this proposed DFR Framework, this server will collect all the logs and information from different components of the framework. This server allows the forensic investigator to select a specific timestamp and create a report including detailed information from all servers in the network. It also supports search functions to help the forensic investigator to search specific information.

5   Evaluation of DFR Framework Artefact

The proposed artefact was evaluated by the subjective method (i.e. by a group of experts).

5.1   Preparation for Evaluation

Based on the evaluation criteria, 18 questions were created and provided to all experts with the proposed framework artefact, descriptions of all system components' functions and supplement reading of related material. In order to thoroughly evaluate the proposed artefact, the following six experts from related fields with exclusive knowledge and work experience were selected and requested to conduct the evaluation of the proposed artefact against the suggested evaluation criteria [48].

5.2   Evaluation of the Artefact

The following group of experts participated in the artefact evaluation.

Expert 1 has specialised in areas such as Health Information Technology (HIT), Wireless Networks, Internet of Things (IoT), and Software Defined Networks (SDN) for more than 25 years. He was a researcher and the head of the management section of Ministry of Science and Technology, Iraq. Currently, he is a senior academic staff member of an Institute of Technology in New Zealand as well as being a certified instructor of Cisco Networking Academy for 14 years.

Expert 2 has been a senior field service engineer for GE Healthcare and Siemens Private Limited (Pte. Ltd) specialising in medical equipment including X-Ray systems, Digital Mammography, Digital Angiography, Computed Tomography (CT) and Magnetic Resonance Imaging (MRI) systems for more than 19 years in the Healthcare Industry.

Expert 3 has extensive knowledge and work experience as a digital forensic investigator and a researcher of more than 7 years. He has also been a lecturer in Information Security, Risk Management, Microsoft Windows Servers based Networks at both graduate and post-graduate level for more than 4 years. Moreover, Expert 3 has published and presented several research papers closely related to the new emerging research areas in Digital Forensics and Network Security at internationally well-recognised conferences and journals.

Expert 4 has more than seven year experience as a Digital Forensic Analyst in the IT Industry. He has worked on hundreds of investigations looking for electronic evidence on a wide range of devices including computers, mobile devices, global positioning system (GPS) units, and other storage devices. For the last two years, Expert 4 has worked as a Penetration Tester, working on a number of security reviews, including web application reviews, mobile application testing and hardware reviews of embedded devices. He has also written a Master's thesis on forensic data collection of Apple iPhones and recently presented a number of disclosed vulnerabilities found in modern routers.

Expert 5 specialises in wireless networks and security, cloud computing, network architectures and protocols and SDN. He is an assistant professor and also a reviewer for many prestige international journals and conferences. Expert 5 used to work as a head of telecommunications and computer networks group for a university.

Expert 6 has extensive experience in Medical Information Systems, Digital Forensics, Cyber Security, Risk Management and Standards of more than 20 years. He is not only a full-professor at a University in New Zealand, but also has been a negotiator representing New Zealand in the International Organization for Standardization and the International Electrotechnical Commission (ISO/IEC) for 14 years. Moreover, he is a board member of Information Systems Audit and Control Association (ISACA, Auckland Chapter).

6   Findings and Discussions

The evaluated artefact is further analysed using a thematical approach in NVIVO. Thematic analysis is a commonly used approach in conducting qualitative data analysis in DS research. Qualitative methodologies aim to explore complex phenomena [48]. They accept multiple realities and have a commitment to identifying an approach to in-depth understanding of the phenomena, a commitment to participants' viewpoints, conducting inquiries with the minimum disruption to the natural context of the phenomenon, and reporting findings in a literary style rich in participant commentaries. Thematic analysis is a process for encoding qualitative information [49]. This type of analysis looks mainly at "what and how" the data say and aims at identifying patterns within the data.

Feedback received from expert evaluations, a central theme was established first which is the DFR framework. The central theme is then categorised into three areas for further analysis against evaluation criteria discussed in Sect. 3 in three system dimensions, which are "Goal", "Environment" and "Structure/Activity". "Goal" is to analyse whether or not the DFR framework has achieved its design goal. "Environment" is to analyse whether or not the DFR framework has been consistent with an organization and its people. "Structure/Activity" is to analyse the artefact's dynamic of operations and its functionalities. Each of these three areas is divided into smaller areas of prospects for in-depth analysis. For example, "Goal" is divided into two smaller areas of prospects of "Efficacy" and "Validity". "Environment" is divided into two smaller areas of prospects of "Consistency with organization" and "Consistency with people". "Consistency with people" is then classified into "Utility", "Understandability" and "Ease of use". "Activity" is divided to "Completeness".

6.1 Word Frequency Analysis Results

Word frequency queries in NVIVO provides researchers with a list of the most frequently occurring words or concepts of referenced material. This can help the researcher in not only identifying possible themes, particularly in the early stages of the project; but also finding the most frequent words occurring in a particular referenced material. Figures 4 and 5 show top 20 most frequent exact word matches and stemmed word matches.

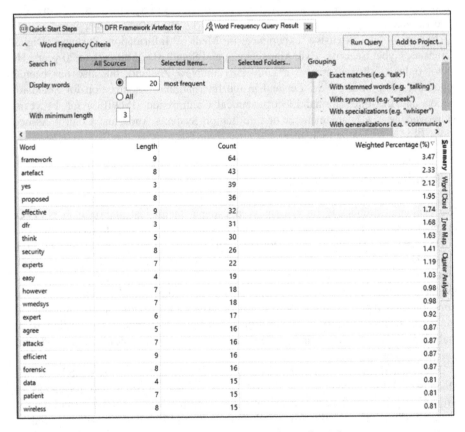

Fig. 4. Top 20 most frequent exact word matches

Comparison is made after running both features to provide more in-depth and broad analysis. Noticeably, "effective" goes up to fourth place on the stemmed word match table (see Fig. 5) from the fifth place on exact word match table (see Fig. 4). Also, "implemented" has gone up. This is consistent with overall experts' comments that emphasize implementing the artefact. Moreover, "use/useful", "efficient/efficiency" and "easy" are also at the top of the table. Thus, analysis shows that experts agree that the proposed DFR framework is "effective", "efficient", "useful" and "easy" to implement and utilise.

After conducting the "word frequency query", a "text search query" is used to understand the meaning of these most frequently appearing words in the content. This can provide the researcher with better understanding of the implication and interpretation of these words in context and with a more meaningful context for reasoning. Based on the results provided from "word frequency query" and evaluation criteria in Sect. 3, the following words are used, which are "effective", "efficient", "useful", "strength", "weakness", "easy", "security", "safety" and "evidence" showed in Figs. 6, 7, 8, 9, 10, 11, 12, 13 and 14 (see Appendix).

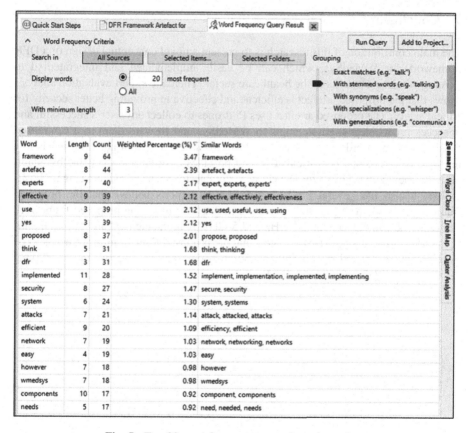

Fig. 5. Top 20 most frequent stemmed word matches

Since the goal of this research is to design and develop a cost-effective DFR framework; hence, "effective" and "efficient" are essential characteristics to evaluate whether or not a such goal has been achieved. The analysis result shows that most of these expert feedbacks provides very positive comments. Thus, the artefact is considered as "effective" and "efficient" in preserving digital "evidence". Consequently, the goal of the study has been achieved. In addition, the artefact is considered as "useful" and realistic in improving and addressing patient "safety" and overall medical system "security" in health clinical environment against attacks. Thus, patient safety is protected and ensured. Additionally, according to the experts, the artefact is easy to implement, understand and use. "strength" and "weakness" analysis show that the proposed DFR framework design is suitable for security risk coverage, has several benefits of "easy" implementation, "easy" to use, low cost resources, and competitive prices. It can also access HL7 and DICOM format. However, the proposed framework does not consider 5 GHz and residual risk management. Otherwise, all experts agree the proposed framework is good in preserving digital evidence and recommend integrating the DFR framework into existing networks in a controlled laboratory environment to prove the concept.

7   Conclusion

The main contribution of this research is to present a novel conceptual design of a DFR framework for WMedSys, which can be easily implemented and integratedlxd to existing wireless networks in the healthcare sector. Thematic expert evaluation analysis shows that the proposed artefact is efficient and effective in providing better security for patient safety. The proposed artefact uses Pi-drones to collect any user's successful and unsuccessful wireless login attempts to WMedSys and forward them to a centralised logging system in order to preserve digital forensic evidence. In addition, it has low resource requirements, is cost-effective and provides customisation benefits by adapting free open-source software. Hence, it is suitable for security risk coverage. Nevertheless, it also has several limitations. Although experts believe that the proposed framework is only designed for WMedSys in 2.4 GHz band, the proposed framework can easily be applied to both 2.4 GHz and 5 GHz by replacing the hardware of the Pi-drone. For future study, experts suggest that the proposed DFR framework needs to be implemented and tested in a controlled laboratory environment to prove this conceptual design of a DFR framework for WMedSys.

Appendix

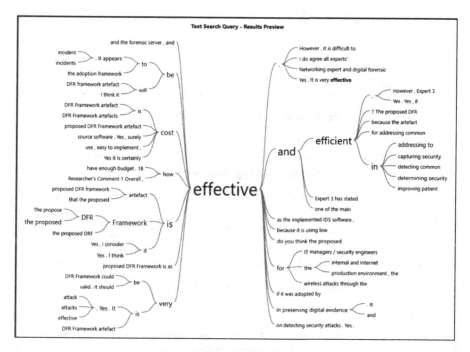

Fig. 6. Text search query result for "effective"

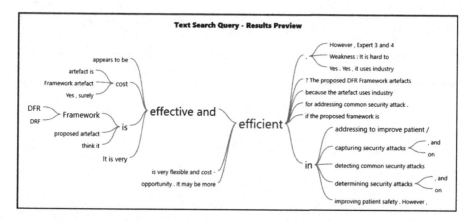

Fig. 7. Text search query result for "efficient"

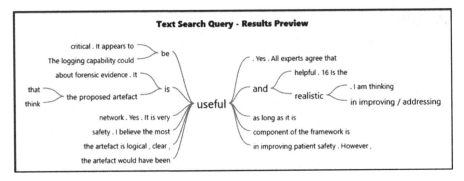

Fig. 8. Text search query result for "useful"

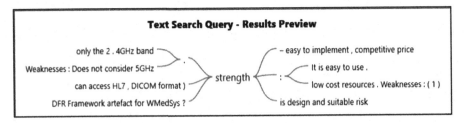

Fig. 9. Text search query result for "strength"

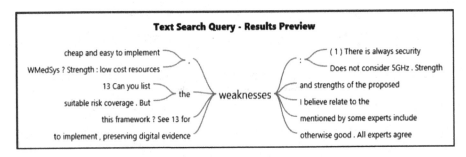

Fig. 10. Text search query result for "weakness"

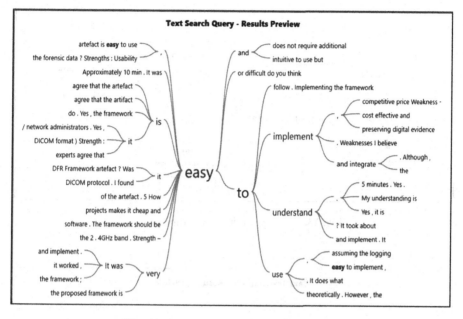

Fig. 11. Text search query result for "easy"

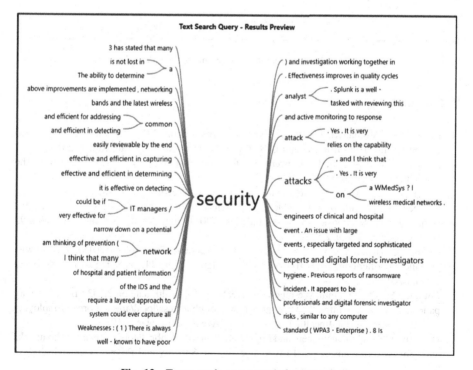

Fig. 12. Text search query result for "security"

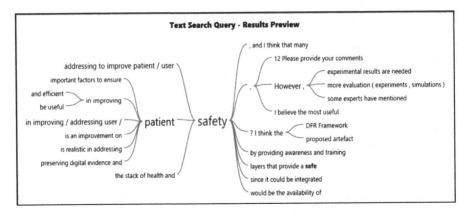

Fig. 13. Text search query result for "safety"

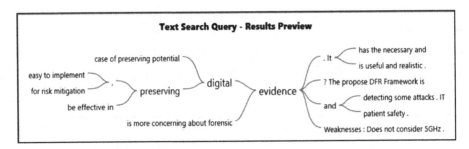

Fig. 14. Text search query result for "evidence"

References

1. Baldoni, R., Montanari, L.: Italian Cyber Security Report 2015 - A national framework. Capienza Università di Roma and CINI Cyber Security National Lab, Roma (2016)
2. Brownlee, N., Guttman, E.: Expectations for Computer Security Incident Response. The Internet Society, Reston (1998)
3. Reggiani, M.: A brief introduction to Forensic Readiness (2016). http://resources. infosecinstitute.com/a-brief-introduction-to-forensic-readiness/#gref. Accessed 13 Mar 2019
4. Napier, J.: NICS forensic readiness guidelines (2011). http://studyres.com/download/4392 801. Accessed 14 Mar 2019
5. Quinn, S.: Hospital pays $55,000 ransom; no patient data stolen (2018). http://www. greenfieldreporter.com/2018/01/16/01162018dr_hancock_health_pays_ransom/.   Accessed 14 Mar 2019
6. Ehlinger, S.: Former employee reportedly steals mental health data on 28,434 Bexar County patients (2017). https://www.expressnews.com/business/local/article/Former-employee-reportedly-steals-mental-health-12405113.php. Accessed 14 Mar 2019
7. Halperin, D., et al.: Pacemakers and implantable cardiac defibrillators: software radio attacks and zero-power defenses. In: IEEE Symposium on Security and Privacy, Oakland (2008)

8. Radcliffe, J.: Hacking Medical Devices for Fun and Insulin: Breaking the Human SCADA System (2011). https://media.blackhat.com/bh-us-11/Radcliffe/BH_US_11_Radcliffe_ Hacking_Medical_Devices_WP.pdf. Accessed 14 Mar 2019

9. Li, C., Zhang, M., Raghunathan, A., Jha, N.K.: Attacking and defending a diabetes therapy system. In: Burleson, W., Carrara, S. (eds.) Security and Privacy for Implantable Medical Devices, pp. 175–193. Springer, New York (2014). https://doi.org/10.1007/978-1-4614-1674-6_8

10. Gollakota, S., Hassanieh, H., Ransford, B., Katabi, D., Fu, K.: They can hear your heartbeats: non-invasive security for implantable medical devices. In: ACM SIGCOMM 2011 Conference, New York, NY (2011)

11. Clark, S.S., Fu, K.: Recent results in computer security for medical devices. In: Nikita, K.S., Lin, J.C., Fotiadis, D.I., Arredondo Waldmeyer, M.-T. (eds.) MobiHealth 2011. LNICST, vol. 83, pp. 111–118. Springer, Heidelberg (2012). https://doi.org/10.1007/978-3-642-29734-2_16

12. Burleson, W., Clark, S.S., Ransford, B., Fu, K.: Design challenges for secure implantable medical devices. In: 49th ACM/EDAC/IEEE Design Automation Conference (DAC), San Francisco (2012)

13. Hermans, J., Tinholt, H.W., de Wit, J.: Achieving digital forensic readiness (2015). https://assets.kpmg.com/content/dam/kpmg/pdf/2016/03/Achieving-Digital-Forensic-Readiness-12 -9-2015.pdf. Accessed 13 Mar 2019

14. Alenezi, A., Hussein, R.K., Walters, R.J., Wills, G.J.: A framework for cloud forensic readiness in organizations. In: 5th IEEE International Conference on Mobile Cloud Computing, Services, and Engineering (MobileCloud), San Francisco (2017)

15. Rahman, N.H., Glisson, W.B., Yang, Y., Choo, K.K.: Forensic-by-design framework for cyber-physical cloud systems. IEEE Cloud Comput. 1(3), 50–59 (2016)

16. Raju, B.K., Geethakumari, G.: An advanced forensic readiness model for the cloud environment. In: International Conference on Computing, Communication and Automation (ICCCA), Noida, India (2016)

17. De Marco, L., Ferrucci, F., Kechadi, M.: Reference architecture for a cloud forensic readiness system. In: EAI Endorsed Transactions on Security and Safety, pp. 1–9 (2014)

18. Kebande, V.R., Venter, H.S.: A cloud forensic readiness model using a Botnet as a Service. In: International Conference on Digital Security and Forensics (DigitalSec2014), Ostrava, Czech Republic (2014)

19. Harbawi, M., Varol, A.: An improved digital evidence acquisition model for the Internet of Things forensic I: a theoretical framework. In: 5th International Symposium on Digital Forensic and Security (ISDFS), Tirgu Mures, Romania (2017)

20. Endicott-Popovsky, B., Frincke, D.A., Taylor, C.A.: A theoretical framework for organizational network forensic readiness. J. Comput. 2(3), 1–11 (2007)

21. Kebande, V.R., Karie, N.M., Venter, H.S.: A generic digital forensic readiness model for BYOD using honeypot technology. In: IST-Africa Week Conference, Durban, South Africa (2016)

22. Kebande, V.R., Karie, N.M., Omeleze, S.: A mobile forensic readiness model aimed at minimising cyber bullying. Int. J. Comput. Appl. 140(1), 28–33 (2016)

23. Barske, D., Stander, A., Jordaan, J.: A digital forensic readiness framework for South African SME's. In: Information Security for South Africa (ISSA), Sandton, Johannesburg, South Africa (2010)

24. Ngobeni, S., Venter, H., Burke, I.: A forensic readiness model for wireless networks. In: Chow, K.-P., Shenoi, S. (eds.) DigitalForensics 2010. IFIPAICT, vol. 337, pp. 107–117. Springer, Heidelberg (2010). https://doi.org/10.1007/978-3-642-15506-2_8

25. Rahman, A.F.A., Ahmad, R., Ramli, S.N.: Forensic readiness for wireless body area network (WBAN) system. In: 16th International Conference on Advanced Communication Technology, Pyeongchang (2014)

26. Cusack, B., Kyaw, A.K.: Forensic readiness for wireless medical systems. In: 10th Australian Digital Forensics Conference, Perth, Western Australia (2012)

27. Ieong, R.S.C.: FORZA – digital forensics investigation framework that incorporate legal issues. Digit. Invest. **3S**, S29–S36 (2006)

28. Reggiani, M.: A brief introduction to Forensic Readiness (2016). https://resources. infosecinstitute.com/a-brief-introduction-to-forensic-readiness/#gref. Accessed 14 Mar 2019

29. Kent, K., Chevalier, S., Grance, T., Dang, H.: NIST Special Publication 800-86: Guide to Integrating Forensic Techniques into Incident Response. National Institute of Standards and Technology, Gaithersburg (2006)

30. Given, L.: The SAGE Encyclopaedia of Qualitative Research Methods. SAGE Publications, London (2008)

31. Kebande, V.R., Venter, H.S.: A functional architecture for cloud forensic readiness large-scale potential evidence analysis. In: 4th European Conference on Cyber Warfare and Security (ECCWS), Hertfordshire, Hatfield (2015)

32. Grobler, C.P., Louwrens, C.P.: Digital forensic readiness as a component of information security best practice. In: Venter, H., Eloff, M., Labuschagne, L., Eloff, J., von Solms, R. (eds.) SEC 2007. IIFIP, vol. 232, pp. 13–24. Springer, Boston, MA (2007). https://doi.org/ 10.1007/978-0-387-72367-9_2

33. Rowlingson, R.: A ten step process for forensic readiness. Int. J. Digit. Evid. **2**(3), 1–28 (2004)

34. Sule, D.: Importance of forensic readiness. ISACA J. **1**(2014), 1–5 (2014)

35. CYFOR: Specialists in Organisational Forensic Readiness Planning and Implementation (2018). http://cyfor.co.uk/digital-forensics/forensic-readiness-planning/. Accessed 13 Mar 2019

36. Makutsoane, M.P., Leonard, A.: A conceptual framework to determine the digital forensic readiness of a Cloud Service Provider. In: Portland International Conference on Management of Engineering & Technology (PICMET), Kanazawa, Japan (2014)

37. Reddy, K., Venter, H.: A forensic framework for handling information privacy incidents. In: Peterson, G., Shenoi, S. (eds.) DigitalForensics 2009. IFIPAICT, vol. 306, pp. 143–155. Springer, Heidelberg (2009). https://doi.org/10.1007/978-3-642-04155-6_11

38. Mouhtaropoulos, A., Dimotikalis, P., Li, C.T.: Applying a digital forensic readiness framework: three case studies. In: IEEE International Conference on Technologies for Homeland Security (HST), Waltham, MA (2013)

39. Kebande, V.R., Ntsamo, H.S., Venter, H.S.: Towards a prototype for achieving digital forensic readiness in the cloud using a distributed NMB solution. In: 15th European Conference on Cyber Warfare and Security (ECCWS), Munich (2016)

40. Kebande, V.R., Venter, H.S.: Requirements for achieving digital forensic readiness in the cloud environment using an NMB solution. In: 11th International Conference on Cyber Warfare and Security, Boston (2016)

41. Mouhtaropoulos, A., Li, C.T., Grobler, M.: Digital forensic readiness: are we there yet? J. Int. Commer. Law Technol. **9**(3), 173–179 (2014)

42. Pooe, A., Labuschagne, L.: Cognitive approaches for digital forensic readiness planning. In: Peterson, G., Shenoi, S. (eds.) DigitalForensics 2013. IFIPAICT, vol. 410, pp. 53–66. Springer, Heidelberg (2013). https://doi.org/10.1007/978-3-642-41148-9_4

43. Ngobeni, S.J., Venter, H.S.: The design of a wireless forensic readiness model (WFRM). In: Information Security South Africa Conference, Johannesburg, South Africa (2009)

44. Lalla, H., Flowerday, S., Sanyamahwe, T., Tarwireyi, P.: A log file digital forensic model. In: 8th International Conference on Digital Forensics (DF), Pretoria, South Africa (2012)
45. Alrajeh, D., Pasquale, L., Nuseibeh, B.: On evidence preservation requirements for forensic-ready systems. In: 11th Joint Meeting on Foundations of Software Engineering, Paderborn (2017)
46. Fleming, R.F.: Towards the analysis of information environment resilience for real enterprises (Doctoral thesis). The University of New South Wales, Canberra, Australia (2010)
47. Peffers, K., Tuunanen, T., Rothenberger, M.A., Chatterjee, S.: A design science research methodology for information systems research. J. Manag. Inf. Syst. 24(3), 45–77 (2007)
48. Vaismoradi, M., Turunen, H., Bondas, T.: Content analysis and thematic analysis: implications for conducting a qualitative descriptive study. Nurs. Health Sci. 15(1), 398–405 (2013)
49. Boyatzis, R.: Transforing Qualitative Information: Thematic Analysis and Code Development. SAGE Publications, Thousand Oaks (1998)

An IoT-Based Healthcare Ecosystem for Home Intelligent Assistant Services in Smart Homes

Miguel Mendonça[1], Tomás Jerónimo[1], Mauro Julião[1], João Santos[1], Nuno Pombo[1], and Bruno M. C. Silva[1,2(✉)]

[1] Instituto de Telecomunicações, Departamento de Informática, Universidade da Beira Interior, Rua Marquês d'Ávila e Bolama, 6201-001 Covilhã, Portugal
miguelbmg@hotmail.com, tomasfjeronimo@gmail.com,
maurojuli@hotmail.com, joaoaaasantos@gmail.com,
ngpombo@ubi.pt, bruno.silva@it.ubi.pt
[2] Universidade Europeia, IADE, Av. D. Carlos I, 4, 1200-649 Lisbon, Portugal

Abstract. Home Intelligent Assistants (HIAs) typically integrate several types of healthcare and well-being solutions that include mobile applications, sensors or wearables. These solutions are usually connected to the HIA through the Internet designing an Internet of Things (IoT) ecosystem. This paper presents an IoT healthcare ecosystem for smart home environments that considers both indoor and outdoor scenarios. The main goal is to monitor in a pervasive way habitant vital signs, such as heart rate, temperature, and respiration, while sleeping or any other indoor and outdoor activity. A breast sensor band and smartwatch were used as wearable sensors of the ecosystem. Furthermore, smartphones and tablets were used has interfaces of the HIA. The service-oriented architecture that integrates all the IoT solutions was constructed and a secure authentication model was implemented to maintain health data privacy. This framework's main goal is to allow the integration of other IoT-based solutions regardless of its hardware or software. The proposed ecosystem and integrated solutions were validated both in terms of features and communication through a series of experiments on real devices through a Wi-Fi network.

Keywords: Health · Mobile health · IoT · Health IoT · Smart home

1 Introduction

With the advent of the Internet of Things (IoT) paradigm new and pervasive communication scenarios arose, creating new business and research opportunities. IoT includes and enables interconnected computers, machines, sensors, other objects and people, each with a unique identifier to transmit information to a network without the need for human interaction. The number of devices capable of being part of one of these systems is increasing, and as a result more and more projects focused on services or applications have been created in order to monitor, using sensors, patients health data that can be used, stored and transmitted to other devices and systems [1, 2]. IoT empowers new types of services that can benefit users in both professional and personal lives. Services, such as, manufacturing [3], transports and logistics [4], healthcare [5], Smart Cities [6], and Smart Homes [7, 8] are examples of field on which IoT is already creating new research and/or business opportunities. IoT is already having a great impact on the health industry. When connected to the Internet, common medical devices can collect and share great amounts of data, enabling a broader view of symptoms, and the possibility of doctors' remote care. IoT devices can help professionals to monitor several health statuses, these technologies include, for example, glucose monitoring pills, connected inhalers to help with diseases such as asthma or diabetes, ingestible sensors. These devices, coupled with a powerful monitoring platform, can certainly improve patients' health and change the way health is currently managed.

Health IoT-based solutions are becoming popular in a healthcare system that is failing all around the world and is already unsustainable. With the growth of the elderly population who spend most of their time at home, there is an urgent need for low-cost and sustainable healthcare solutions. One solution is to transform the normal home into a ubiquitous computing technology environment that supports the care and well-being of the elderly living independently. These home systems are called smart homes and are currently a hot research topic [9]. This concept involves the use of technology to ensure more comfort and safety. The first step to home automation is an Internet system. IoT networks and Smart Homes are undoubtedly unseparated. The network is responsible for connecting all smart devices, usually to Home Intelligent Assistants (HIAs) that integrate several types of devices that include mobile applications, sensors or wearables. Wi-Fi and Bluetooth are the best-known home networking technologies, but they won't always be the most efficient. Wi-Fi consumes too much power, and Bluetooth can only be used in small places. Although the great potential, IoT networking, and smart home environments raise critical challenges such as security, data value but mainly interoperability [10, 11].

This paper presents an IoT healthcare ecosystem for smart home environments. This work main goal is to present a framework for real-time monitoring, that allows the integration of both indoor and outdoor solutions, through a service-oriented architecture, called HIAS. This ecosystem includes two IoT-based solutions. The indoor solution monitors heart rate and respiration while sleeping or resting on a couch through a breast sensor band. The outdoor solutions react to emergency scenarios and monitors in real-time the heart rate, temperature and location of the user through a smartphone and a smartwatch. The HIA service-oriented architecture that integrates all the IoT solutions has also a secure authentication model that was specifically implemented for these scenarios to maintain health data privacy. This work aims to resolve both security and interoperability issues, that are common on these networks and solutions. The HIAS was already designed thinking on interoperability and the presented solutions were constructed for different users, scenarios, and environments. For this first version of the IoT ecosystem, the presented cloud architecture and integrated solutions were validated through a series of experiments on real devices through a Wi-Fi network. The proposed IoT ecosystem for both indoor and outdoor scenarios is presented in Fig. 1. It includes the following applications:

- A HIAS application that integrates all functionalities and respective interfaces.
- A mobile application for a smartwatch that collects in real-time user health data, such as, heart rate and temperature.

- A mobile application for smartphones that allows a user to initiate an emergency wi-fi call or warning to healthcare professionals or familiars through the HIAS services.
- A web application that receives a wi-fi call from the emergency mobile application. This web solution includes geo-location in real-time and voice recognition algorithms.
- A mobile application that collects health data from wearable sensors, specifically a chest band, and forwards it to the HIAS server.

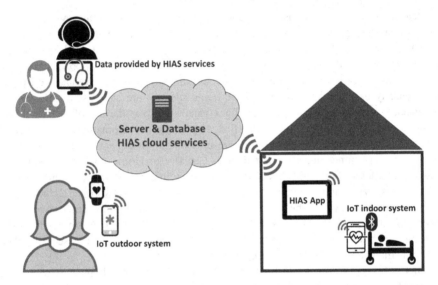

Fig. 1. System architecture of the proposed IoT-based healthcare ecosystem for home intelligent assistant services in smart homes

The remainder of this paper is organized as follows. Section 2 presents a review of the related work in both healthcare IoT and smart home solutions. In Sect. 3, the IoT healthcare ecosystem cloud architecture is presented its security mechanisms. Section 4 presents the indoor solution and its implementation details. The construction and implementation of the IoT outdoor solution are presented in Sect. 5. Finally, the paper is concluded in Sect. 6 and future work is presented.

2   Related Work

IoT solutions can provide several advantages to services provided by the health industry. On the one hand, the use of sensors allows health providers to monitor the patient's vital signs and the use of smart devices can help to transmit that information across medical facilities [12, 13]. On the other hand, IoT may support health providers by reducing various monotonous tasks and/or to enable alerts in case of emergency [14]. The CareAngel platform [15] provides a service to, remotely, monitor the health condition of elderly people. This is achieved through the use of artificial intelligence and speech recognition. The service allows his users to do daily calls to a virtual assistant, where some information about their condition is collected. This information is then shared with the authorized agents like family members or health providers. Several clinics and hospitals already use this innovative platform, however, there are some limitations associated with it, especially the resistance to change from pen-and-paper to digital technology. Apple Watch Healthcare [16] is another service integrated into a smartwatch device and uses sensors to monitor his user's heart health. Afterward, these data are processed aiming to provide valuable information about the user's condition and to emit alerts whenever an unusual heart rate value is detected. In the smart home industry, applications that act like home intelligent assistants, controlling home sensors or actuators are becoming very popular. The Wink [17] and the Samsung SmartThings [18] are currently the most popular hubs on the market. Both have their applications in leading application stores. These hubs allow the integration of smart systems and other devices and the manipulation of them all through a mobile device. Washing machines, refrigerators, vacuum cleaners, lamps, irrigation sprinklers, air conditioning are some examples of smart devices that can be easily controlled. These hubs have an architecture that can integrate new devices, however, this process is not always flexible. In smart home environments or IoT networks, data-related issues, such as storage, retrieval, processing, and security, are major concerns. These systems usually adopt cloud computing architectures that must be designed and developed taking into consideration these issues and the integration of third-party applications [19].

2.1 Contributions

The presented work gathers contributions from the above study. When compared with other solutions presented in the literature, the system proposed in this paper differs from them because it offers a service-based architecture, called HIAS, prepared for the integration of third-party applications with a security model for user and data privacy. Moreover, this ecosystem for smart homes considers not only indoor solutions but also outdoor applications that interact with the HIAS. Moreover, the HIAS ecosystem creates ubiquitous communication scenarios where persons can be constantly monitored. The next sections will present the HIAS architecture and integrated solutions in detail.

3 HIAS Cloud Architecture and Security Implementation Details

This section presents the design and implementation details related to the cloud architecture of the IoT-based healthcare ecosystem and the security mechanisms implemented. This service-oriented architecture, called HIAS, was design with three main requisites: (1) Easy integration of new users, applications or other devices, such as, sensors and actuators; (2) the ecosystem should consider indoor and outdoor scenarios, including mobility environments; and (3) All health data and user authentication should be private and secure.

3.1 HIAS Service Based Architecture

The HIAS system architecture is an model-view-controller (MVC) architecture, and so there are three main pillars, which are:

- Model: The main component of the architecture execution. This is responsible for modeling, storage, retrieval and process data.
- View: The purpose of the view is to present to clients all the information presented in the system. It is the user interface layer.
- Controller: This layer receives information and data that interprets, changes if necessary, and sends to the model.

All clients (users, devices, etc.) communicate with the HIAS through HTTP requests and HTTP responses, and all information is exchanged between the server and clients in JSON format, a simple and fast format. This system is also present in the models. Data models are responsible for aggregating and matching all acquired data. The view is responsible for sending and receiving the data. The view does not care about the data types or how they are acquired, it is only limited to visually presenting the result. In this case, it is responsible to send information for applications that complete this system. All services that are part of the controller add, update, extract or read data from the database. These services were developed in an ASP .NET Core Web Application in C#, which offers object-oriented programming and freedom to interact with other software developed in other programming languages. Figure 2 describes the HIAS service-based oriented architecture. Each service has an associated HTTP request link. Then each customer selects the services they want to use and links them to the source code of the software they are developing. Since HIAS is a service-based architecture, services are the main pillars of the whole system. As mentioned earlier, and to integrate various applications and software into one architecture, the services were developed aiming at to allow CRUD operations on data. To read the information present in the database is used the GET method. This method was chosen because it does not allow the modification of the data.

To add and update the data, the POST method is used. Requests using this method are never cached and do not remain in the browser history, which ensures high security for this system. These POST requests have no data length restrictions, which allows large data to be used by this method. One such example is the electrocardiographic readings, which is a fairly long list of data but is saved from the database without any problem.

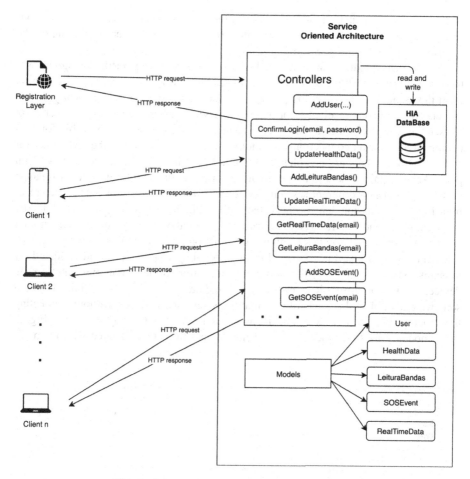

Fig. 2. IoT ecosystem service-based architecture.

All of these services make a direct connection to the database and, depending on what they do, execute SQL commands to manipulate or query information. Finally, add and update services return a flag depending on the execution of the command - success or failure flag. There is also in this system a single registration layer for all applications: the user will only need to register once and will be able to login to all applications that are part of this universe. This is because there is a unique database shareable between all applications.

3.2 HIAS Security Mechanisms

The constructed and implemented security procedures' main goal are to increase communication security between systems while decreasing their development time. These processes can be handled by dedicated modules. These modules are bundled with the systems and are responsible for producing secure and privacy-oriented communication channels between the constituents of the ecosystem. As such, constituents of this system do not communicate directly with each other, depending on the security modules to produce communications.

The security modules are composed of a public-key pair, a certificate signed by a trusted authority and three different services responsible for (1) receiving information from the associated device. This process consists of a service running locally on the associated device that receives information the device wishes to send over the network; (2) sending information to another security module. A service is responsible for producing an SSL socket connection with another security module using the certificates for authentication. Afterward, an ephemeral public-key pair is produced and an ephemeral public key (its pair) is sent to the receiving security module. With this, a key exchange protocol produces a different session key for each transmission sent over the connection. Each transmission sent is encrypted with a unique session key using public-key cryptography.; and (3) receiving information from the security module of another device. A service that handles receiving information sent by another security module. The data that is received is decrypted using public-key cryptography and validated for transmission errors. If valid, the now decrypted information is communicated to the device, for it to perform whatever function is required. The security modules function somewhat as a black-box, where information is sent and received without it affecting the structure and inner workings of the associated devices. Has may be seen in Fig. 3, these modules are fairly independent of the devices that are associated with them.

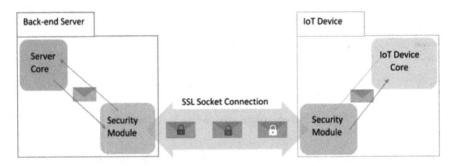

Fig. 3. Representation of the ecosystem security procedures and its modularity.

Development, maintenance, and updates of these modules can be performed in separate of the IoT solutions. By having several abstractions on the architecture of the system to allow for these modules to work associated with the IoT devices, only minor changes to the security modules are be needed for them to function in different IoT devices and systems. As a result, development times of security solutions can be cut down because of the increased interoperability of different devices or systems with the security modules. This increasing focus on the development of a smaller number of security solutions instead of a dedicated security solution for each device or system, possibly resulting in an overall boost in solution quality.

4 IoT Solution for Outdoor Emergency Scenarios

This section presents an IoT solution integrated into the HIAS, for outdoor scenarios, specifically for emergencies. This solution's main goal is to react and facilitate the communication between users and the emergency services, through the HIAS system. This solution is able to monitor his user's health status and location and send this information in real-time to the HIAS. In case of an emergency, and if the user is unable to contact by himself the emergency services, the home intelligent system will contact them automatically (or a familiar). This IoT solution also includes a voice recognition application that enables a faster reaction and action from the caretaker. This application can be used by a familiar, through the HIAS, or a third-party client, such as an emergency service operator. Therefore, as may be seen in Fig. 4, this outdoor IoT solution includes three different applications, a smartwatch application, a mobile application, and an operator application. A security module, named MD BARS, was also implemented and it's integrated with the HIAS security procedures.

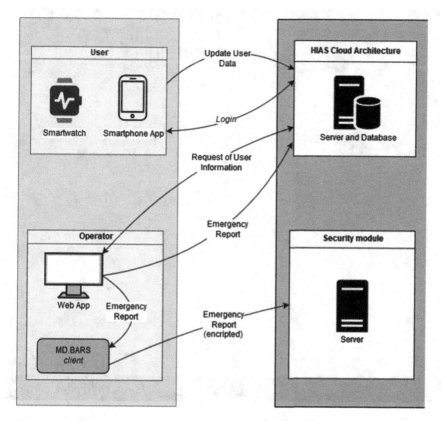

Fig. 4. System architecture design of the outdoor IoT solution for emergency scenarios

The smartwatch application has the objective of providing the system with real-time data about his user's heart rate and body temperature, by using the sensors integrated into the device. At the same time, the app should be able to detect any dangerous values and automatically trigger an emergency request. The collected data is then transferred to the smartphone application (Fig. 4) where his user can it will be processed and presented to the user in graphical form. Besides that, the mobile app also allows the user to login to his HIA account and edit his personal and health information (Fig. 5b). Information such as the user's age, health condition, and medical history can also be valuable to the emergency agents, however, it is a hugely time-consuming task to describe them with accuracy in a stressful scenario. The final piece of information collected by the mobile application is the device location. The app takes advantage of the powerful GPS, that the majority of modern smartphones possesses, to provide accurate data about his user's location and, in case of an emergency, collects real-time updates about it. To start an emergency call, all the user has to do is access the application and press the button on the center of the screen (Fig. 5a). This will trigger two actions: first, a request will be sent to the central server, informing that an emergency call has been initiated, and at the same time, a call to the predefined emergency number will be triggered.

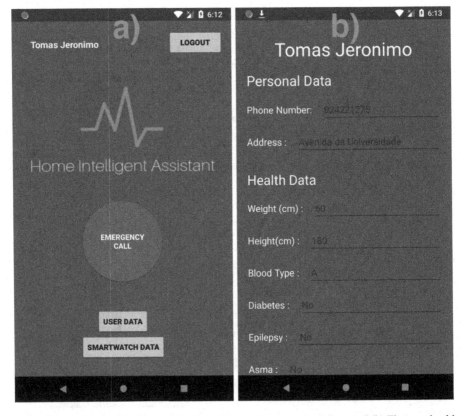

Fig. 5. Smartphone application interface. (a) The main activity interface; and (b) The user health information interface.

The final application of the outdoor IoT solution that is integrated with the HIAS is a web application, and it can be seen in Fig. 6. This application can be used by emergency operators, or informal caretakers (friends or familiars) through the HIAS. The main goal of this application is to provide them with the most relevant information about each situation, reducing to reduce the time required to evaluate each emergency call and deploy the appropriate rescue agents. In order to achieve this, at the beginning of the call, the application will immediately present the user's heart rate, body temperature, and location. This will give the operator some basic information about the user's situation and health status before the conversation between them even starts. Then, during the call, the operator's voice will be processed using a speech recognition algorithm to detect whenever he requests new information. These requests are then processed by the application that tries to respond with the data at his disposal. After the end of the call, the operator is required to give a summary of the situation, and this will be sent to the central server, and added to the user's history.

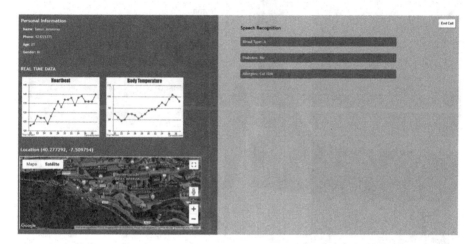

Fig. 6. Emergency web application of the outdoor IoT solution. Interface displayed in the HIAS application.

The communication between these three applications is only possible because of the HIA service where they are integrated, where a central server and database allows the exchange of information among them. The communication protocols between each application and the central server were developed to allow secure data exchange and maintain user's privacy.

5 IoT Solution for Indoor Monitoring Scenarios

This section presents an IoT solution integrated into the HIAS, for indoor scenarios. This solution allows us to monitor in real-time the user's heartbeat and respiration while sleeping, resting, sitting on a chair or couch through the support of biometric sensors, specifically through a chest band (Fig. 7a). This chest band is a research product developed by PLUX [20]. A mobile application (Fig. 7b) was constructed and used as a gateway for relay data from the sensors to the HIAS, through the Internet.

However, communication between the sensors and the smartphone is made via Bluetooth. While wearing the chest band, the user or a familiar start the mobile application that will collect, process and send the data to the HIAS, for storage and analysis. This solution was constructed and aims the detection and prevention of the activation of the autonomic nervous system while sleeping. However, it can be used in other indoor scenarios. The only requirement is that users should not be in movement around the house. One possible scenario is the real-time monitoring of habitants' heartbeat and respiration while watching TV or reading a book.

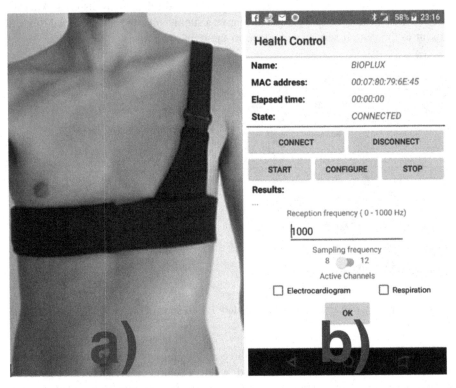

Fig. 7. (a) Chest Band used for health data collection; and (b) mobile application to collect and forward user data from sensor to the HIAS

Considering the above scenarios, when the application starts will be required authentication data, so, if the user is not registered in the HIAS system, he can perform the registration, and after, perform the login, so that a unique user can access all functionalities and store his biometric data, or visualize his past acquisitions. The mobile device must support the use of Bluetooth since the chest band connects to the mobile via Bluetooth, and, in case it doesn't have, the user will only be presented with limited functionalities, such as a list of previous acquisitions and analysis of preliminary ECG and Respiration graphs. The communication between the device and the chest band can occur in the classic Bluetooth connection or using Bluetooth Low Energy. As there is a possibility that there are several chest bands in the area, it must be selected of the list the desired one comparing the presented MAC address on the screen with the one registered on the band. This application allows the user to select the acquisition parameters such as Reception Frequency and Sampling Frequency, defining the accuracy of the receive data and presentation of the graphs. It already has standard values if the user doesn't want to change them. On acquisition mode, the data sent by the Bluetooth device are received asynchronously by the mobile device and then sent to the local broadcast receiver, using a specific object.

After all the health data is collected, it is sent to the HIAS integrated database through HTTP requests being stored for posterior visualization. This data consists of three columns, being the first the total milliseconds of acquisition, the second and the third is the value of ECG and respiration at a given time respectively. The ECG works detecting and assigning values to the electrical signals generated by the heart. Respiration is obtained indirectly, by measuring body volume changes such a thoracic circumference. For this to work is was used as an API developed by Plux company that can be found at their website [20], which consists of a jar file containing all the API object code. As mentioned earlier, this application allows data visualization from a past biometric acquisition. For this purpose, the application performs a request to the database allowing the user to select the desired one from a list sorted by date. After the selection, another request to the database is made so, it can return the data to populate the graphs and calculate the values of heart and respiration rate values (Fig. 8). Based on sex, age, and weight, if a certain biometric acquisition has abnormal ECG or respiration value, a notification is triggered informing the user and advising him to visit a health professional.

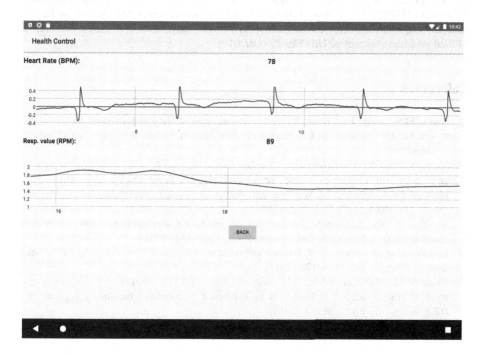

Fig. 8. Heart rate and respiration values displayed in the HIAS application.

6   Conclusions and Future Work

This paper presented an IoT-based healthcare ecosystem for Home Intelligent Assistant Services in Smart Homes. This work main goal consists of real-time monitoring and reaction to hazards situations through the integration of IoT solutions for indoor and outdoor scenarios on a Home Intelligent Assistant, called HIAS. It considers three main components: a modular service-oriented architecture, an indoor system for biofeedback monitoring while sleeping or resting and an outdoor emergency call/react system. Moreover, a module for secure authentication and privacy was constructed and implemented. The presented ecosystem includes the use of mobile devices and wearable sensors. It is very easy to use in terms of design and usability. Although is not focused on elderly people, it requires a small interaction among users and devices. This ecosystem architecture was constructed and implemented, considering the interoperability challenges that these networks usually have. Therefore, the system is prepared to integrate other third-party solutions.

As future works, experiments with real users to evaluate the correct operation of this ecosystem will be performed, considering the users' satisfaction and usability. Furthermore, it will consider the integration of more applications within this framework. The main future goals for this ecosystem are advanced interoperability and security research.

Acknowledgements. Contributing to this work, the authors affiliated with the Instituto de Telecomunicações also acknowledge the funding for this research: the FCT/MEC through national funds and when applicable co-funded by FEDER – PT2020 partnership agreement under the project UID/EEA/50008/2019. (Este trabalho é financiado pela FCT/MEC através de fundos nacionais e quando aplicável cofinanciado pelo FEDER, no âmbito do Acordo de Parceria PT2020 no âmbito do projeto UID/EEA/50008/2019).

References

1. Uddin, M.S., Alam, J.B., Banu, S.: Real time patient monitoring system based on internet of things. In: 4th International Conference on Advances in Electrical Engineering (ICAEE), p. 516 (2017)
2. Andriopoulou, F., Orphanoudakis, T., Dagiuklas, T.: IoTA: IoT automated sip-based emergency call triggering system for general eHealth purposes. In: 2017 IEEE 13th International Conference on Wireless and Mobile Computing, Networking and Communications (WiMob), pp. 362–369 (2017)
3. Bi, Z., Da Xu, L., Wang, C.: Internet of things for enterprise systems of modern manufacturing. IEEE Trans. Ind. Inform. **10**(2), 1537–1546 (2014)
4. Liu, W., Gao, Z.: Study on IOT based architecture of logistics service supply. Int. J. Grid Distrib. Comput. **7**(1), 169–178 (2014)
5. Alam, M.M., Malik, H., Khan, M.I., Pardy, T., Kuusik, A., Le Moullec, Y.: A survey on the roles of communication technologies in IoT-based personalized healthcare applications. IEEE Access. **6**, 36611–36631 (2018)

6. Du, R., Santi, P., Xiao, M., Vasilakos, A.V., Fischione, C.: The sensable city: a survey on the deployment and management for smart city monitoring. IEEE Commun. Surv. Tutor. **21** (2), 1533–1560 (2019)
7. Suryadevara, N., Mukhopadhyay, S.C.: Smart Homes Design, Implementation and Issues (2015). https://doi.org/10.1007/978-3-319-13557-1_1
8. Ahlgren, B., Hidell, M., Ngai, E.C.: Internet of things for smart cities: interoperability and open data. IEEE Internet Comput. **20**(6), 52–56 (2016)
9. Pouryazdan, M., Kantarci, B.: The smart citizen factor in trustworthy smart city crowdsensing. IT Prof. **18**(4), 26–33 (2016)
10. Li, W., Logenthiran, T., Phan, V., Woo, W.L.: A novel smart energy theft system (SETS) for IoT-based smart home. IEEE Internet Things J. **6**(3), 5531–5539 (2019)
11. Park, E., Cho, Y., Han, J., Kwon, S.J.: Comprehensive approaches to user acceptance of internet of things in a smart home environment. IEEE Internet Things J. **4**(6), 2342–2350 (2017)
12. Wan, J., Al-Awlaqi, M., Li, M., O'Grady, M., Gu, X., Cao, N.: Wearable IoT enabled real-time health monitoring system. EURASIP J. Wirel. Commun. Netw. 298 (2018)
13. Satija, U., Ramkumar, B., Sabarimalai, M.: Real-time signal quality aware ECG telemetry system for IoT-based health care monitoring. IEEE Internet Things J. **4**(3), 815–823 (2017)
14. Uddin, M., Alam, J., Banu, S.: Real time patient monitoring system based on internet of things. In: 4th International Conference on Advances in Electrical Engineering (ICAEE), Dhaka, Bangladesh, 28–30 September 2017, p. 516 (2017)
15. CareAngel. Virtual Nurse Assitant. https://www.careangel.com/. Accessed 22 June 2019
16. Apple. Healthcare-Apple Watch - Apple. https://www.apple.com/healthcare/apple-watch/. Accessed 22 June 2019
17. Wink. https://www.wink.com/about/. Accessed 22 June 2019
18. Samsung SmartThings. https://www.samsung.com/us/smart-home/. Accessed 22 June 2019
19. Mokhtari, G., Anvari-Moghaddam, A., Zhang, Q.: A new layered architecture for future big data-driven smart homes. IEEE Access **7**, 19002–19012 (2019)
20. PLUX. Wireless biosignals. https://plux.info/. Accessed 1 July 2019

Author Index

Printed in the United States
By Bookmasters